Now That You've Lost It

Other books by Joyce D. Nash

Maximize Your Body Potential

Taking Charge of Your Smoking

Binge No More: Your Guide to Overcoming Disordered Eating

The New Maximize Your Body Potential

Now That You've Lost It

How to Maintain Your Best Weight

Joyce D. Nash, Ph.D.

toExcel

San Jose New York Lincoln Shanghai

Now That You've Lost It
How to Maintain Your Best Weight

Published by toExcel
an imprint of iUniverse.com, Inc.

For information address:
iUniverse.com, Inc.
620 North 48th Street
Suite 201
Lincoln, NE 68504-3467
www.iuniverse.com

Originally published by Bull Publishing Company

ISBN: 0-595-00387-7

Printed in the United States of America

Table of Contents

Preface

Most people who get to goal weight confirm that losing weight was easy compared to the challenge of keeping it off. People can and do lose weight—but most of them regain it. Experts have learned a lot about what is needed to help people lose weight. Now efforts are turning to the problem of backsliding. It appears that keeping the weight off involves something different than what is involved in losing it in the first place.

More and more research is pointing to the involvement of cognitive factors—thinking—in successful, long-term weight management. Although changing thinking has been included as one component of many behavioral weight loss programs, it has been hypothesized that cognitive coping may be most relevant for successful maintenance.

This seems particularly true because so much of relapse is instigated or accompanied by painful emotions. Emotions and thinking go together. If you can learn to manage your thinking, your ability to cope with painful emotions will be significantly improved.

Likewise, relapse is often facilitated by environmental situations—going out to dinner with friends, having an argument with someone, being bored with nothing to do, or just having attractive food readily available.

This book was written primarily for the person who has reached goal weight or is close, and now faces the challenge of keeping it off. It is also appropriate for those people who are in the early phases of a weight loss effort, but who are looking ahead to the future. It is never too soon to learn how to overcome backsliding.

Chapter 1, *The Big Challenge: Keeping It Off,* provides an overview of what factors contribute to relapse, as well as what is known to ensure long-term weight management success. In particular, the role of thinking and how it relates to staying at goal weight is considered.

Motivation for weight control depends upon the stage of change you are in. Chapter 2, *Balancing The Pros and Cons,* invites you to assess your level of motivation, and take steps to increase it if necessary.

Chapter 3, *Learning To "Think Smart"*, describes the process of thinking and the factors that can undermine successful maintenance. Different types of distorted thinking, called "thinking traps," as well as irrational beliefs and negative expectations, all can undo motivation and promote a return to old habits. Suggestions are given on how to get out of such traps and change negative beliefs and expectations.

In particular, increasing positive self-talk and decreasing negative self-talk is important for maintaining success. Chapter 4, *Using Self-talk Effectively*, introduces the concept of the "golden ratio"—the notion that it is the particular *balance* of positive to negative self-talk that counts. Techniques for altering this balance are provided in this chapter.

In Chapter 5, *Coping With Social Influences*, the focus changes to environmental factors that contribute to backsliding. How other people help or hurt your efforts is considered, and suggestions are given for taking charge of these influences.

Being able to create and maintain satisfying relationships is a crucial factor in both the mental and physical health of all human beings—and it is important for weight control as well. Chapter 6, *Improving Your Relationships*, is devoted to helping you learn how to do just this. First, the basics of a healthy relationship are described. Suggestions are then given for building intimacy in relationships, communicating effectively, and managing interpersonal conflict.

Emotions play an important role in weight management success. Chapter 7, *Overcoming Depression and Anxiety*, and Chapter 8, *Managing Anger and Loneliness*, both provide a better understanding of what produces these emotions, and what you can do to cope with them more effectively.

A particular challenge, especially for the dieter who succeeds in reaching goal weight by rigidly controlling what she eats, is binge eating. Chapter 9, *Coping With Binge Eating*, describes this problem and gives specific suggestions for overcoming it.

Chapter 10, *Overcoming Backsliding*, draws on the research that has investigated how relapse can be prevented. This chapter describes how high risk or crisis situations contribute to backsliding, and gives suggestions for coping more effectively with them. Errors in thinking are again addressed, this time in the context of relapse. The need to adjust your lifestyle so that backsliding is less likely is also covered.

Increasingly, obesity is being seen as a chronic problem that cannot be adequately addressed in a brief intervention of only 10 or 20 weeks. Staying at goal weight requires ongoing support. Sometimes this support is most appropriately in the form of psychotherapy. Or it may mean participating in a formal weight maintenance program. Chapter 11, *Reaching Out For Help*, assists you in deciding what kind of additional support you might need, and how to reach out and get it.

Finally, Chapter 12, *Coping With Success,* helps you decide what is a healthy weight for you—one that you can live with. Additional factors that undermine success are considered, and suggestions are given for coping with situations such as: other people's expectations of you now that you are at goal weight, your own tendency to continue to think of yourself as fat even though you aren't any more, and your fear of regaining the weight.

Throughout this book you will find a variety of self-tests and exercises. These are intended to help increase your personal awareness and self-understanding of the factors that might get in the way of your long-term success. Feel free to disregard the results of a given self-test if it doesn't seem to fit for you. But take the time to fill them out and do the exercises suggested. By doing so you will increase your chances of success.

Increased awareness and self-understanding are a necessary first step that enables you to find a solution that works for you. Ultimately, you need to discover the factors that are most likely to undermine your success, and to design a solution for appropriate action to overcome these problems.

Many people participated in the development of this book, not the least of which were my clients over the years who taught me so much about weight management. In particular, I owe the idea for the book, and the instigation to write it, to David Bull, my publisher and editor. All those who participated in the review of this book as well as my former book, ***Maximize Your Body Potential,*** which served as the basis for this book, also deserve another thank you. Thanks also goes to Covert Bailey and Albert Stunkard, MD, for their endorsements. Finally, my husband Morgan White was patient and supportive throughout the long hours I spent working at the computer and leaving him to his own devices.

It is my sincere hope that this effort will benefit those who have made the monumental effort to reach goal weight, and want to stay there.

J. D. N.

Chapter 1

The Big Challenge: Keeping It Off

AFTER REGAINING ALL of the 67 pounds she lost, the well-known talk show host Oprah Winfrey declared, "I'll never diet again!" Dieters nationwide could empathize with her experience.

During her progress toward a thinner self, her fans watched with a mixture of joy and apprehension. They celebrated with her when she triumphantly announced that she had reached her goal weight. And as they detected the relentless return of unwanted pounds, no doubt they were painfully reminded of their own losing battles with weight control.

The lose-it-and-gain-it-all-back-and-more experience is all too common for most dieters. Few actually get to goal weight, and of those who do, most relapse. However, some dieters have a greater risk of relapse than others.

For instance, severely obese dieters, who use a supplemented fast but who don't get in and stay in a group program that helps them change their eating behavior, almost always fail to maintain the weight they lose. If they do get group counseling, about a third will reach their target weight. The chances of maintaining goal weight are increased if they then participate in the maintenance phase of the program.[1,2] Even so, only 30% of women and 58% of men have been found to be within 10 pounds of goal weight 18 months later.

Most moderately overweight dieters who lose weight in behavioral programs of short duration—lasting from 10 to 20 weeks—experience the yo-yo syndrome of regaining and losing the weight again. Allowing for this up-again down-again pattern, less than 3% of men and 29% of women were found to be at or below the reduced weight they attained in the program, when measured again four years later.[3]

What Causes Relapse?

Why, after all the effort and suffering that goes into losing weight, do dieters "let" themselves regain?

1

Rarely does anyone consciously want to regain weight. Relapse is an insidious process. The returning pounds seem to sneak back, until one day the dieter discovers that most, if not all of the pounds she worked so hard to lose have been regained.

In a story in *People* magazine, Oprah attributed her relapse to "not handling stress properly," and to her early childhood sexual abuse. Although these factors may well have had an influence, *People* noted other important contributors to Oprah's putting back the pounds. She dropped out of her diet group, "kissed off" her maintenance program, stopped exercising, and returned to her old eating patterns. That, of course, is a sure-fire formula for regaining weight.

Still, it doesn't answer the real question of *why*? Shouldn't looking and feeling terrific be enough motivation to maintain a reduced weight? Why do most people who reach goal weight stop doing the very things that work to keep weight off—managing, so to speak, to snatch failure from the jaws of success?

What can the at-goal dieter do to prevent self-defeating habits from returning? To answer these questions, it is helpful to consider what contributes to a weight problem—what "goes against" the dieter's chances of maintaining goal weight—and what it takes to succeed long-term.

Determinants of Body Weight
Eating Too Much

Popular wisdom holds that obesity is simply the result of eating too much, and the best exercise a person can get is to push herself away from the table. There is a certain truth in this. If energy intake exceeds energy expenditure over a long period of time, weight will increase.

But research has not been able to clearly establish that the obese do indeed eat more than the nonobese! Rather, the *kinds* of food that the obese eat—the composition of their diet—is an important clue to what causes and maintains obesity. Eating too much dietary fat (no more than 30% of total calories should be fat calories) appears to be a more important determinant of body weight than the absolute number of calories taken in.[4] But there is more to the story.

Genetic Factors

Recent research has also shown that there is an important genetic component involved in the determination of body weight.[5,6] Heredity can go against the dieter by producing either a lower-than-normal basal metabolic rate (BMR) or a blunted thermogenesis. Together, BMR and thermogenesis account for the energy used by the body to maintain body temperature and to support the activity of the internal organs, but does not include energy needed for physical activity.

Basal Metabolic Rate

Basal metabolic rate, or BMR, is the minimum level of energy required by the body simply to stay alive while completely at rest but without having eaten. For the average sedentary adult, BMR accounts for about 65-75% of total energy expenditure.[7] A lower-than-normal BMR means that fewer than average calories are needed for basic body maintenance.

Thermogenesis

Thermogenesis involves the production of body heat, and is the energy expended by a person over and above BMR, not counting physical activity. It is the energy used to digest food, experience emotional arousal, and raise body temperature in response to cold. Thermogenesis is also increased by the use of stimulants such as caffeine or nicotine. If thermogenesis is blunted, the person uses fewer calories for these needs. All together, thermogenesis is thought to account for about 10% of total energy expenditure.

Studies suggest that BMR may be lower for those who are at risk of developing obesity, and may be a factor promoting weight gain.[4] In addition, BMR has been found to be 10% lower for dieters trying to maintain goal weight than for their lean, non-dieting counterparts.

The evidence for the influence of thermogenesis on the risk of developing obesity or regaining weight lost is not as strong as it is for BMR. Still, there are indications that a significant number of obese people have a lower-than-normal thermogenesis— which could contribute to a weight problem.

Physical Activity

Physical activity accounts for the rest of the energy used by the body after BMR and thermogenesis have been considered. It has been well demonstrated that the obese tend to be less physically active than the nonobese. The trouble is, research has not been able to establish conclusively which comes first. It may be that obese people don't exercise much because of their obesity! Indeed, the severely obese often have to lose weight first in order to begin to exercise.

Most experts emphasize the importance of increasing physical activity as a means of reducing and maintaining a lower body weight. In the average sedentary person, physical activity accounts for 15-20% of the total energy expenditure.[8] When activity is increased—either by undertaking a program of regular exercise or by increasing ordinary daily activity—this percentage, and the number of calories spent, increases.

Increasing physical activity is the only means of getting rid of excess calories that is truly under the control of the person. Getting more exercise also raises metabolic rate and keeps it boosted for a time after exercising is completed. Nearly all of those who have succeeded in maintaining their best weight over the long run have increased their physical activity. Succeeders find a way to make exercise a regular and permanent part of their lifestyle.

Psychological Factors

There are other non-physiological factors that may be going against the dieter's efforts as well. Dr. Judith Rodin at Yale University and her colleagues have proposed one possible model for how psychological factors can place someone at risk for obesity.[9] They proposed that such people are more sensitive and vulnerable than others to certain kinds of arousal.

When confronted with greater and greater stress, or when the problems of life get to be too much for them, the obese-prone tend to eat as a means of coping. People with a weight problem also are prone to eat to self-medicate themselves for physical or emotional pain. Depression, anxiety, and anger have been the emotions reported as the most likely to result in emotional eating, though loneliness and boredom are not far behind. Indeed, interpersonal conflict and difficulties in relationships are strongly associated with stress, negative emotions, and relapse.[10,11,12]

When food is readily available or especially attractive, most people can't resist, but people at risk for obesity are even more vulnerable. They can have a particular problem with the siren call of beautiful food presented at festive social occasions, especially if they have no strategies for coping.

Others argue that dieting itself is the problem—that "diets don't work," and the real issue is self-acceptance regardless of what one weighs. This is the basis for the "fat is beautiful" movement. This notion deserves further consideration.

Rigid Dieting

Research suggests that chronic dieters are those who seem to do really well losing weight and are often the superstars in a weight control program. These "restrained eaters" succeed by rigidly dieting and controlling their eating, at least for a while. However, once they break their diet with even a small slip, this rigid restraint is disrupted and binge eating ensues. If this happens while they are still in a weight control program, the restrained dieter is likely to drop out.

But even if a rigid dieter succeeds in reaching goal weight, failure is likely to be waiting in the wings. Despite short-term effectiveness, rigid dieting eventually produces binge eating, and with it an end to the dieting effort, and subsequent regaining of lost weight.[13,14,15,16,17]

In short, rigid dieting doesn't work. However, the alternative need not be giving up all efforts at weight management. There is a better way, and the odds of achieving long-term success are much better if a good diet is followed flexibly.

Trauma and Stress

Finally, Oprah may be right. Traumatic experiences, especially physical, emotional, or sexual abuse in childhood, can be contributing factors. Although there is little research evidence linking traumatic experiences with overeating or obesity, there is enough anecdotal evidence and data based on clinical experience to warrant giving this notion further consideration.

Dr. Eliana Gil, who specializes in treating victims of abuse, documented the patterns of symptoms in the clients she saw between 1978 and 1986.[18] Overall, her data indicated that nearly one out of five abuse survivors suffers from obesity. Survivors most likely to have such weight problems were those whose abuse began prior to the age of nine.

Most professionals who have worked with the obese for some time recognize that for some people, there is more to their weight problem than simply bad eating habits. Eating is one way of self-medicating, to push away painful memories in consciousness, or the free-floating anxiety that can exist when the memories are still in the subconscious.

Eating is also a way of distracting oneself from present-day problems or a chronically stressful situation. Whether the trauma is in the past, or there is ongoing stress, if these contributors to a weight problem are not addressed, long-term success may be elusive.

Beating the Odds

So, considering all of these hurdles for the would-be weight controller, how is it that some people do succeed, seemingly "against all odds?" Despite discouraging success rates for reaching and maintaining goal weight, the possibility of genetic vulnerability, and the influence of a variety of psychological and social factors, there *are* instances of people who have managed to lose weight and keep it off for many years.[3]

Somehow, these successful maintainers have been able to cope with powerful factors that make them vulnerable to obesity. They have been able to maintain an energy balance that keeps them at their best weight. How are they able to do this? Research tells us that those who succeed long-term make some important and permanent changes in their behavior and thinking—changes that make all the difference.

Factors Associated with Long-Term Success

One of the most important changes associated with long-term success is making regular exercise a permanent part of one's lifestyle. In one study of men and women who used a variety of methods to lose at least 20% of their body weight, and who kept it off for at least two years, the common denominator for all of them was sticking to a program of exercise after reaching goal weight.[19] Research has repeatedly confirmed the critical role that exercise plays in successful maintenance.[20]

Maintaining a controlled level of calories on a day-to-day basis has also been found to be crucial. Those who continue to use the weight control skills they learned in treatment—such as weighing themselves regularly, keeping track of calories or eating behavior, and using problem solving skills—also have a better chance of maintaining weight over the long run.[3] Other factors that seem to help include enrolling in further weight-loss programs, continuing in a formal maintenance program, or staying in contact with a therapist. Such on-going efforts help the at-goal dieter maintain vigilance and awareness of weight fluctuations and thus be able to take corrective action when it is needed.

Another helpful practice is to establish a smaller margin of error as a signal for when to take action. Research has found that people who regarded themselves as overweight when they went more than three pounds over their personally-chosen goal weight had better long-term success than those who gave themselves more latitude.[21]

Surprisingly, gender is a factor in weight loss success. Men seem to lose weight more easily, more quickly, and with fewer complications during treatment than do women. However, when allowance is made for the fact that men are naturally heavier than women to start with, men and women have been found to be equally successful in losing weight.[22]

But the real test is keeping it off, and that's where women actually excel. Not right away—but over time, women do better than men. In a study in which clients who participated in a behavioral weight control program were weighed every year for five years, it was found that, while both men and women tended steadily to gain back weight lost, by the third year of follow-up, women were maintaining better than men.[3] Although men lost more weight than women, both in absolute terms and as a percent of initial body weight, they regained weight faster than women.

Knowing What to Do Doesn't Mean Doing It

Most people understand that increasing exercise, keeping down the number of calories (and especially the fat calories) in the diet, and continuing to use techniques such as self-monitoring and problem solving skills are all necessary for long-term weight control success. But knowing what to do and doing it can be two different things.

Why is it so hard to do what we know perfectly well works? More and more, the experts are coming to suspect that the way the dieter *thinks* has a lot to do with how she behaves! The beliefs she holds about herself and her weight, the expectations she has about her ability to lose weight and maintain success, her expectations for what being thinner will bring, how much attention she devotes to managing herself, the thinking errors she falls prey to, and what she says to herself, all influence her eating and the other behaviors that ultimately affect weight.[23]

Thinking: The Key to Success

Beliefs

Research is beginning to indicate how thinking can influence weight control success. One study compared the beliefs of obese and nonobese women.[24] It was found that the obese tend to reject the idea of self-control and the need to set limits on themselves. Their beliefs might lead to thoughts such as, "Why do I have to watch everything I eat while other people can eat anything they want and not gain weight?"

The obese also are likely to deny the possibility of change. "I guess I'm just meant to be fat." Or, "What with having to run after three children, I can't possibly be expected to manage my weight too." And, "I don't have time right now to try to manage my weight; it's all I can do to manage my job responsibilities."

They often avoid direct expression of feelings, especially anger, preferring instead to "stuff" these feelings. Feelings of being vulnerable or responsible for others are also prevalent, but rarely given a voice: "I shouldn't feel angry." "I can't trust anyone." "If I don't do it, no one else will."

The obese tend to be hard workers who strive for achievement, frequently without sufficient recognition. They usually react to their own failures with guilt and self-recrimination. They may secretly admonish themselves: "I don't deserve to be thin." Their inability to express their feelings can generate conflict and tension in interpersonal relationships, which in turn can lead to overeating.

The kinds of beliefs that typify people who are not very successful in managing weight are those that involve not wanting to set limits or exercise self-control, doubting one's ability to change, rejecting the right to express one's feelings or to speak up for one's needs, desiring to avoid interpersonal conflict, setting up unrealistic expectations for oneself or others, and judging oneself or others harshly.

The conclusion of the researchers carrying out the study was that diets cannot have the desired effect as long as there is no change in these kinds of beliefs, because such beliefs ultimately undermine success.

Self-Confidence

On the other hand, people who have a high level of self-confidence in their ability to lose weight and maintain weight loss, and who believe that what happens is related more to what they do than to some external factor, tend to experience greater and longer-lasting weight control success.

Conversely, people who externalize blame and don't take personal responsibility currently for managing their weight, who blame others or circumstances for their weight problem, or who have a low level of self-confidence in their weight management abilities tend not to undertake a weight management effort, or if they do, they don't do well and may even quit prematurely.

Such "externalizers" are especially vulnerable to any apparently new diet or weight loss program that comes along. The novelty of such a diet or program, or the reported "scientific breakthroughs" often touted for them, brings a sudden rebirth of hope. Ultimately, however, as their lack of *personal* self-confidence reasserts itself, these new efforts are once again doomed to failure.

How can a person increase her self-confidence in the face of repeated weight control failures? First, she needs to decide that something is different now—that something has changed. Whereas in the past, some crucial ingredient for success was missing, now that ingredient is present.

What is different now is that she has learned that she must think differently and do things differently in order to succeed. She must take charge, not only of her behavior, but also of her thinking.

In addition to developing a new mental perspective, the dieter needs some concrete evidence to boost her self-confidence. It has been said that "nothing helps success more than success." That is, those who start a weight control effort and experience early success in losing weight tend to develop more and more self-confidence.

Again, those with greater self-confidence do better, and for that, early success is important. The person who puts in more effort in the beginning of a weight control effort, and creates some early success for herself provides momentum likely to carry her through to sustained success.

Of course, success is relative. What is success to one person may not be success to another. One person's two pound weight loss success over the past week may be another's perceived failure. Not only must a person actually lose weight in order to build initial self-confidence, the person must *perceive* the weight loss as a success and give herself credit for it.

How do we know that self-confidence is so important? In one study, 414 Weight Watchers' members were telephoned weekly for 12 weeks and asked to rate both their self-confidence about reaching goal weight and their perceived success to date.[25] Those who eventually dropped out over the 12-week period tended to give lower weekly self-confidence ratings and to perceive themselves as less successful, even though there was no difference between their weight losses and that of the members who stayed. The researchers concluded that dropouts had doubts about reaching goal weight long before they actually dropped out, and further, that their perception of success, more than actual success, influenced their decision.

What about self-confidence after goal weight has been achieved? Presumably the person reaching goal weight feels pretty triumphant and self-confident. Even Oprah was confident enough to declare to her fans when she hit her goal that she would never let herself be fat again. Sometimes *overconfidence*, together with the desire to get all that pain and effort behind her, can lead the newly successful dieter to forsake the vigilance and self-awareness necessary to stay at goal weight. To counter this tendency, Weight Watchers used to tell its at-goal members, "Always remember: You are a fat person in a thin body."

How does one keep up self-confidence during maintenance? Basically you must do what it takes to be successful in losing weight: Accept personal responsibility for what you eat and do, avoid externalizing blame; and just as important, notice and give yourself credit for the small, day-to-day successes. Each time you engage in exercise, mentally pat yourself on the back. Each time you make a healthy food choice, feel proud of your healthier eating habits.

Outcome Expectancies

A high level of self-confidence in one's ability to change is not enough, however. What one expects to have happen or how one thinks things will improve as a result of reaching goal weight is also important.

Although some people undertake a weight reduction effort for health reasons, most people do so because they want to look better and feel more attractive. But what happens to the person who reaches goal weight and doesn't judge herself to be as attractive as she had hoped to be? The disappointment can lead to eating to feel better—and subsequent regaining of the weight lost.

In a revealing study, researchers investigated the arguments for (pro) and against (con), that a person might make in deciding to undertake or maintain a weight control effort.[26] An example of a pro argument would be, "I would feel sexier if I lost weight," a con argument, "I won't be able to eat the foods I like."

The researchers found that people still thinking about undertaking a weight control effort could think of a lot of both pro and con arguments. On the other hand, once they started a weight control effort, they thought primarily of the pro arguments and seemed to have "forgotten" about the unpleasant aspects of trying to lose weight. Finally, however, when they got to the maintenance phase, they were again conscious of both the pro and the con arguments.

It seems that once a weight control effort is undertaken, the tendency is to idealize the outcome, in order to maintain the effort it takes to lose weight. But once goal weight is reached, reality sets in again.

There are on-going costs to maintaining the new, lower weight. It is necessary to keep on exercising and to eat differently than before. Not only are the costs once again salient, the expected rewards—feeling more attractive or sexy, getting the approval of one's family, or having better relationships— may not be fully realized. Or the rewards may not really outweigh the costs.

The point is to be realistic about what one can expect as a result of getting to goal weight. The person who gets to goal weight is likely to be just a smaller version of her old self. She will likely have the same old job, the same old spouse, and the same old worries. She *may* feel better about herself, but she will not be 22 years old again. She *may* gain increased admiration from others, but if she doesn't have her own self-acceptance, this attention may be difficult to handle. With all this unaccustomed attention, she may get the feeling that the rules have changed but no one has told her what the new rules are.

Whether the rewards of being thinner are enough to balance the costs that must be paid to stay that way is purely a subjective matter. How a person chooses to view herself and her situation is what counts. Recognizing and accepting the pros and cons ahead of time, and being realistic about what getting to goal weight can bring, will inoculate the dieter against disappointment later—and increase her chances of staying at goal weight, because she won't fall into the trap of thinking that goal weight will magically make her happier.

Awareness

Self-control requires self-focused attention.[27] That is, in order to exercise self-control in anything, one has to be aware of one's behavior, and simultaneously must compare this behavior to some relevant standard. The aim is to bring the two into alignment. Thus, writing down what is eaten each time one eats something is a powerful behavior change technique, because it forces the dieter to be conscious of what and how much she is eating relative to the number of calories she needs to restrict herself to daily in order to lose weight.

Eating is a behavior that can easily be put on "automatic pilot." As such, little conscious control is required, and food choices are made on the basis of habit or preferences of the moment. By going on automatic pilot, one avoids potentially uncomfortable decision-making about food. Any critical evaluation of what to eat in order to lose or maintain weight is suspended. In addition, such "unconscious" eating may help to numb out painful feelings or to distract attention from problems and difficulties.

When a person writes down what she eats before eating it, she is more likely to question her choices and behaviors. By thus going off automatic pilot, she may also have to confront painful feelings associated with other problems in her life. She may come full face with what she had been trying to avoid by eating on automatic pilot. Self-focused attention directed to food and eating behavior inevitably raises awareness of *other* areas of one's life—including areas that may be painful.

Those who are successful in managing their weight in the long-term have developed the ability to tolerate the possible discomfort that can come from increased self-focus. Or they have used this new-found self-awareness to deal more effectively with those things that are causing pain.

Perhaps they have learned to be more assertive, or to manage conflict more effectively. Those who find the pain too great to deal with, or who don't learn new ways to respond, tend to back away from self-focused attention. As a result, careful self-monitoring is eventually discontinued, leading ultimately to self-regulatory failure.

How one is doing socially is also important. In order to improve self-control and increase chances for long-term success, it is necessary to develop effective skills in communication and in managing interpersonal relationships. The better one is in this regard, the more smoothly things will go with others. When relationships are going relatively well, increased self-focused attention will not present undue discomfort.

It is important then to be able to maintain awareness and self-focused attention during the maintenance phase of weight control. This is why continuing to participate in additional weight control programs or maintaining regular contact with a therapist contributes to on-going success. Such pursuits assist people to stay focused on managing weight.

Distorted Reasoning

Failures in eating behavior are often preceded by certain kinds of reasoning that lead to problems. One kind of faulty thinking involves the use of rationalizations that allow a person to break her diet. For example, "I've had such a stressful day; I deserve a little treat." When the logical outcome of a thought is to overeat, some kind of distorted reasoning is involved.[28]

Another type of distorted reasoning involves rigid thinking. Dieters who frequently lose control over their eating tend to use "rigid control," whereas dieters who rarely lose control tend to think more flexibly. Rigid control is characterized by "black-and-white," "all-or-nothing" thinking. Either the rigid dieter never touches the "wrong" foods, or a single bite of a forbidden food means all further effort is useless because clearly "I can't do it."

Chronic rigid dieters tend to diet frequently and count calories, but do not use such behavioral strategies as taking small helpings or eating slowly. They worry a lot about what they weigh, but they do not pay much attention to changes in their weight or figure—until the problem is well out of hand. They put a lot of effort into resisting temptation, but if they do succumb, they often fail to compensate by eating less or getting more exercise shortly after their indiscretion.

Table 1.1

"Negative" and "Positive" Self Talk

Negative or self-defeating self-talk

Rigid thinking: This includes all-or-none self-statements and thoughts which suggest overly restrictive comparisons of the self, extreme evaluations, perfectionistic goals, and excessive expectations for the self. Such thoughts tend to reflect extreme dieting or excessive effort.

Thoughts reflecting issues of self-control: Thoughts in this category include not wanting to set limitations on oneself, choosing not to exert self-control, or feeling out-of-control or unable to exert control. Acting without thinking or forethought, or choosing to ignore the consequences of one's actions, so that there is a lapse in control, or feeling confused about how one's actions contribute to outcomes, also suggests problems with self-control.

Self-punishing thoughts: Thoughts of this type reflect guilt, self-blame, self-denigration, anger directed at the self, or excessive self-criticism that demoralizes rather than empowers. Included are thoughts that dwell on failures or focus excessively on painful or unpleasant feelings that lead one to feel immobilixed or moved to self-defeating action.

Positive or coping self-talk

Flexible thinking: These thoughts reflect balanced comparisons, even-handed evaluations, and matter-of-degree explanations for dietary slips or personal failures. Such thoughts reflect the setting of realistic and attainable goals and not being too hard on oneself without also rationalizing inappropriate behavior.

Self-instructional thoughts: These what-to-do and how-to-cope thoughts focus on what actions need to be taken to facilitate movement toward a goal. Such thoughts may reflect genuine problem solving efforts or attempts at decision-making. They may call attention to the need to use behavioral weight control techniques or the need to "get back on track" with weight management efforts. Sometimes these thoughts seem to sound "parental" or self-critical, but the effect is stern support rather than destructive demoralization.

Self-reinforcing thoughts: This category includes pats-on-the-back thoughts and thoughts that call the person's attention to successful actions that facilitate goal achievement. Such thoughts may note what one has learned from an experience, or may call attention to the supportive behavior of others toward oneself. These thoughts acknowledge to oneself one's accomplishments, progress, strengths, or good qualities.

Other kinds of distorted reasoning include making excessive and inappropriate connections between one's self-esteem, weight, approval from others, and self-control efforts.[29] Self-esteem related thoughts appear to underpin the "fear of weight gain" idea that is central to eating disorders of all kinds.

Self-Talk

Self-talk is simply the "little voice in the head" that most people recognize as their own, commenting on their behavior and circumstances in general. Some people worry that admitting they talk to themselves is tantamount to

Table 1.1

"Negative" and "Positive" Self Talk *(continued)*

Negative or self-defeating self-talk

Negative expectancies: Thoughts in this category focus on doubts about one's ability to change, to lose weight, to keep it off, or to recover from relapse. The result is that self-confidence declines. Included here are thoughts focusing on arguments against managing weight, without balancing such thoughts with arguments in favor of trying. Thus, one expects not to be able to lose weight or to keep it off.

Ambivalent or Avoidance Thoughts: Thoughts in this category reflect ambivalence about using a proven weight management technique. Or such thoughts may suggest that the person avoids doing something that can support weight control, such as asserting herself or expressing her feelings appropriately. Such thoughts may reflect conflict avoidance, passivity, or difficulty standing up for oneself.

Rationalizations and excuses: Included here are thoughts excusing inappropriate behavior or suggesting reasons why it would be okay to behave in ways that make weight management more difficult. Also included in this category are thoughts that blame other people, heredity, stress, or "unchangeable" factors for one's failure to manage weight successfully. Thoughts that involve denial or that are self-deluding are included in this category.

Positive or coping self-talk

Positive expectancies: These include self-confident thoughts that one can handle a situation, recover from a slip, continue to lose weight successfully, or stay at goal weight. Thoughts in this category may also reflect realistic evaluations about how being thinner will change one's experience. Or, such thoughts may present a balanced view of the arguments for and against weight management.

Assertiveness and coping skills: These thoughts reflect the ability to cope with stressful situations, to get one's needs met, or to express difficult feelings appropriately. Such thoughts may also suggest one who is willing or able to get the support of others. Thoughts in this category may also suggest a belief that self-focused attention is necessary and appropriate for success.

Thoughts reflecting goals, values, or ideals: Thoughts in this category reflect higher-level, more abstract, or more distant goals, or abstract principles, values, and ideals. Examples would include reminding oneself of wanting to get to goal weight, wanting to attain improved health or some other benefit. Such thoughts might remind oneself of having personal responsibility for or control over actions and outcomes.

an admission of being crazy. In fact, all people—crazy and sane alike—talk to themselves. The difference is that sane people know it is their own voice. Crazy people think it's someone else's voice.

There are two kinds of self-talk. "Negative" self-talk is any kind of thought that undermines a person's progress. Such self-talk may refer to unrealistic or perfectionistic goals or self-doubts. Often such a thought feels self-punishing, self-critical, or self-blaming, but sometimes it feels "good"—at least initially. An example is when one thinks of an excuse to overeat—only later to feel bad about the behavior. If the thought hinders coping behavior and inhibits goal achievement, it is self-defeating or "negative."

"Positive" self-talk, on the other hand, is a coping thought and facilitates achievement of a goal. Such self-talk may take the form of instructions about what to do or how to cope. At other times positive self-talk involves giving oneself mental pats on the back or reminders of what one wants eventually to achieve. Usually such self-talk feels good, but sometimes it can have a critical or "parental" tone such as, "Okay, stop fooling around and get on the exercise bike now."

The various categories of negative and positive self-talk are presented in Table 1.1. Twelve categories, grouped by complementary pairs, describe the characteristics for each pole of the negative/positive dimension of self-talk.

Balance of "Negative" and "Positive" Self-Talk

In trying to help people cope better, some have advocated learning to think only positive thoughts. Norman Vincent Peale was one of the best known champions of the power of positive thinking. Others, such as Albert Ellis, have advocated focusing attention solely on uncovering, challenging, and eliminating negative thoughts.

It would be quite unrealistic to expect that a person think only positive, coping thoughts. Such a person would seem very Pollyanna-ish and out of touch with reality. Likewise, a person who only thought negative, self-defeating thoughts would probably be seriously mentally ill. In fact, all people engage in both positive and negative self-talk. The ratio of positive to negative thoughts is what is really important.

People whose negative, self-defeating self-talk outweighs their positive, coping thoughts tend not to do well in their weight management efforts. To attain success, the objective is to get the positive self-talk to outweigh the negative, aiming for a ratio of about 2 to 1, positive to negative. Although there is no way to measure a person's actual ratio of positive and negative weight-related thoughts, one can apply the general prescription for learning to think "smart"—namely to increase the positive and decrease the negative.

In general, the person who has a greater chance of achieving long-term weight management success will engage in more self-talk that reflects flexible thinking, how-to-cope thoughts, pats-on-the-back thoughts, more self-confident thoughts, and thoughts reflecting assertiveness and coping skills. Conversely, the dieter with the greatest chance of failure will engage in more self-talk that reflects rigid thinking, struggles with self-control, self-denigration, self-doubt and unrealistic expectancies, and excessive ambivalence or avoidance.

Prescription for Long-Term Success

Thinking "smart" is only one part of the solution, but it is a critical part. Thinking smart is the basis for those changes which ultimately make the difference—making exercise a permanent part of one's lifestyle; limiting overall calories, but particularly fat calories; continuing to use the behavioral techniques that work (e.g., keeping track of what one eats); and developing skills for coping with stress and having healthy relationships. In some cases, the solution may also include therapy for dealing with past traumatic experiences or ongoing stressful situations.

Professionals and lay people alike must begin to recognize that obesity is a chronic condition. It is not simply the result of bad eating habits that have been learned, although this is often part of the problem. It is not a symptom of some personality problem or mental condition, although these may coexist with the obesity.

Obesity is a lifestyle problem. It involves behavior and thinking, and it exists in a social as well as a personal context. Staying at one's best weight requires a strategy of lifelong weight management that need not be obsessive or overwhelming. Rather, maintaining goal weight needs to be seen as a kind of personal hygiene routine—something one devotes regular but minimal attention to *every day,* much as one brushes one's teeth daily.

Summary

In the chapters that follow, the reader will learn how to talk herself into success, think "smart," relate better to others, cope with painful emotions, better manage binge eating, overcome backsliding, reach out for additional help, and cope with success.

This book is a guide for the reader to use in finding and implementing her own solution—her own personal weight hygiene routine. It is likely to take a while before such a routine feels "normal," but eventually, successful weight management can be as automatic—and painless—as brushing one's teeth.

References

1.   Wadden, T.A., & Stunkard, A.J. (1986). Controlled trial of very low calorie diet, behavior therapy, and their combination in the treatment of obesity. *Journal of Consulting and Clinical Psychology, 54,* 482–488.

2.   Kirschner, M.A., Schneider, G., Ertel, N.H., & Gorman, J. (1988). An eight-year experience with a very-low-calorie formula diet for control of major obesity. *International Journal of Obesity, 12,* 69–80.

3.   Kramer, F.M., Jeffery, R.W., Forster, J.L., & Snell, M.K. (1989). Long-term follow-up of behavioral treatment for obesity: Patterns of weight regain among men and women. *International Journal of Obesity, 13,* 123–136.

4.   Shah, M., & Jeffery, R.W. (1991). Is obesity due to overeating and inactivity, or to a defective metabolic rate? A review. *Annals of Behavioral Medicine, 13,* 73–81.

5.   Stunkard, A.J., Foch, T.T., & Hrubec, Z.A. (1986). A twin study of human obesity. *Journal of the American Medical Association, 256,* 51–54.

6.   Stunkard, A.J., Sorensen, T.I.A., Hanis, C., Teasdale, T.W., Chakraborty, R., Schull, W.H., & Schulsinger, F. (1986). An adoption study of human obesity. *New England Journal of Medicine, 314,* 193–198.

7.   Jequier, E. (1984). Energy expenditure in obesity. *Clinical Endocrinology and Metabolism, 13,* 563-580.

8.   Garrow, J.S. (1974). *Energy Balance and Obesity in Man.* New York: Elsevier.

9.   Rodin, J., Schank, D., Striegel-Moore, R. (1989). Psychological features of obesity. *Medical Clinics of North America, 73,* 47–66.

10.   Cummings, C., Gordon, J.R., & Marlatt, G.A. (1980). Relapse: Prevention and prediction. In W.R. Miller (Ed.), *The Addictive Disorders: Treatment of Alcoholism, Drug Abuse, Smoking, and Obesity.* (pp. 291–322). New York: Pergamon.

11.   Hafner, R.J., Rogers, J., & Watts, J. McK. (1990). Psychological status before and after gastric restriction as predictors of weight loss in the morbidly obese. *Journal of Psychosomatic Research, 34,* 295–302.

12.   Stalonas, P.M., Perri, M.G., & Kerzner, A.B. (1984). Do behavioral treatments of obesity last? A five-year follow-up investigation. *Addictive Behaviors, 9,* 175–183.

13.   Gormally, J., Black, S., Daston, S., & Rardin, D. (1982). The assessment of binge eating severity among obese persons. *Addictive Behaviors, 7,* 47–55.

14.   Gormally, J., Rardin, D., & Black, S. (1980). Correlates of successful response to a behavioral weight control clinic. *Journal of Counseling Psychology, 27,* 179–191.

15.   Keefe, P.H., Wyshogrod, D., Weingerger, E., & Agras, W.S. (1984). binge eating and outcome of behavioral treatment of obesity: A preliminary report. *Behavior Research and Therapy, 22,* 319–321.

16.   Marcus, M.D., Wing, R.R., & Hopkins, J. (1988). Obese binge eaters: Affect, cognitions, and response to behavioral weight control. *Journal of Consulting and Clinical Psychology, 56,* 433–439.

17.   Marcus, M.D., Wing, R.R., & Lamparski, D.M. (1985). Binge eating and dietary restraint in obese patients. *Addictive Behaviors, 10,* 163–168.

18.   Gil, E. (1988). *Treatment of Adult Survivors of Childhood Abuse.* Walnut Creek, CA: Launch Press.

19.   Colvin, R.H., & Olson, S.B. (1983). A descriptive analysis of men and women who have lost significant weight and are highly successful at maintaining the loss. *Addictive Behaviors, 8,* 287–295.

20.   Westover, S.A., & Lanyon, R.I. (1990). The maintenance of weight loss after behavioral treatment. *Behavior Modification, 14,* 123–137.

21.   Stuart, R.B., & Guire, K. (1978). Some correlates of the maintenance of weight lost through behavior modifications. *International Journal of Obesity, 2,* 225–235.

22.   Forster, J.L., & Jeffery, R.W., (1986). Gender differences related to weight history, eating patterns, efficacy expectations, self-esteem, and weight loss among participants in a weight reduction program. *Addictive Behaviors, 11,* 141–147.

23.   Nash, J.D. (1991). *Cognition and Obesity: Development and Validation of a Weight Control Cognitions Questionnaire.* Unpublished doctoral dissertation. Pacific Graduate School of Psychology, Palo Alto, CA.

24.   Kreitler, S., & Chemerinski, A. (1988). The cognitive orientation of obesity. *International Journal of Obesity, 12,* 403–415.

25.   Mitchell, C., & Stuart, R.B. (1984). Effect of self-efficacy on dropout from obesity treatment. *Journal of Consulting and Clinical Psychology, 52,* 1100–1101.

26.   O'Connell, D., & Velicer, W.F. (1989). A decisional balance measure and the stages of change model for weight loss. *International Journal of the Addictions, 23,* 729–750.

27.   Ingram, R.E. (1990). Self-focused attention in clinical disorders: Review and a conceptual model. *Psychological Bulletin, 107,* 156–176.

28.   Westenhoefer, J. (1991). Dietary restraint and disinhibition: Is restraint a homogenous construct? *Appetite, 16,* 45–55.

29. Mizes, J.S., & Klesges, R.C. (1989). Validity, reliability, and factor structure of the anorectic cognitions questionnaire. *Addictive Behaviors, 14,* 589–594.

Chapter 2

Balancing the Pros and Cons of Weight Management

ANYONE WHO HAS undertaken a serious weight reduction effort knows that before the dieting actually begins, there is often a period of soul searching. "Do I weigh too much? Should I try now? What should I do? What are my chances of success? What if I fail?"

During this time of contemplation, the would-be dieter struggles with a mental balance sheet of anticipated gains (or benefits) and projected losses (or costs) that might be expected from undertaking such an effort. The decision to go ahead turns on whether the projected overall benefits outweigh the costs. .

What is less well understood is that once a plan of action is initiated, this mental balance sheet changes as a result of the dieter's progress. Whereas would-be dieters experience considerable conflict about whether or not to begin a diet, once the decision is made, new dieters often become euphoric at the beginning of a dieting effort. All they can think about is how wonderful it will be once they reach goal weight. The benefits of losing weight are now at the forefront, and the expected costs seem to have disappeared.

If the dieter starts losing weight as soon as she begins an effort, and if she is happy with how much she is losing, her "happy thinking" may continue for a time. The longer the dieting effort continues, however, the harder it becomes to keep up the effort. The very real costs—such as having to restrict calories and make time for exercise—intrude more and more into consciousness. If the rate of weight loss slows down, and becomes unsatisfactory, the costs tend to loom larger and larger, until they finally overwhelm the hoped-for rewards. At this point, the dieter quits, having lost faith in being able to attain the expected benefits.

The same mental balance sheet of benefits and costs applies to the maintenance stage of weight control. The at-goal dieter must again struggle

18

both with arguments for (pro) and against (con) continuing the effort to stay at goal weight.[1] Now, however, the question is not whether to initiate action, but whether to continue the action already begun.

In many cases, this means continuing efforts to manage weight while perhaps not getting all that was anticipated. That is, the dieter may not feel especially sexy or more attractive, or may not get as much approval from loved ones as she wants, despite having reached goal weight. Upon reconsideration, the balance may have shifted so that the benefits hardly outweigh the costs, if they do at all. When this happens, continued effort to maintain goal weight is in jeopardy.

Balancing the Benefits and Costs

People have a variety of reasons for wanting to lose weight. Most often, they just want to look and feel more attractive. Sometimes they anticipate health benefits. In other cases, they fear losing their job or getting even fatter if they don't act. In most cases, the benefits they expect are things that give pleasure or satisfaction. Sometimes, the benefit is being able to avoid something unpleasant.

In deciding whether to begin a dieting effort, people also anticipate certain costs—having to do something they don't especially want to do or give up something they like. They will have to forego high-calorie foods and won't be able to eat what they want. They will have to exercise self-control. They may have to make time for regular exercise.

Of course, not bothering to lose or control weight also has its costs—decreasing self-esteem and self-approval, continued or increasing disapproval from others, and the possibility of deteriorating health with additional weight gain. The costs of not managing weight are often the stick that drives a weight loss effort.

Sometimes the costs and benefits involved are not so obvious. Food may be used more or less unconsciously to avoid feeling lonely or bored, and its loss as a coping mechanism can send weight management efforts into a tail spin. Increased attention from the opposite sex, or the higher expectations that are placed on the dieter who is now slimmer, may be more of a cost than a benefit, especially if such attentions or expectations cause discomfort.

When the benefits of a particular course of action outweigh the costs involved, a person tends to keep doing whatever produces the rewards. Conversely, a person is prone to stop doing whatever produces punishment or displeasure, or costs more time and effort than the benefits seem worth.

Since both benefits and costs are involved in every behavior pattern—whether it involves eating, exercise, or some other area of life—trade-offs are made between costs and benefits. For example, exercising may provide the immediate benefits of feeling good, and the long-term benefits of improved cardiovascular fitness. But it also takes time that a person might prefer to spend differently, and in the beginning at least, exercise may involve some discomfort. On the other hand, if feeling good after exercise, or wanting to ensure long-term cardiovascular health are perceived as sufficiently valuable, the dieter may be more willing to pay the costs involved, including making time for it and putting out the effort.

The person who exercises regularly usually has a long list of benefits she gets from exercising—feeling good, more energy, ability to eat practically anything she wants, and so forth. If asked what she doesn't like about exercise, she is likely to minimize those aspects. She exercises regularly because for her, the benefits are more apparent than the costs. On the other hand, the person who used to exercise now and then, but doesn't any more, is more likely to give you a long list of the costs of exercise, and to minimize the benefits.

Exactly what constitutes a cost or a benefit depends on one's point of view. What is rewarding to one person may be punishing to another. The benefits to be gotten, or the costs to be paid are what the person thinks they are, not what someone else judges them to be.

If there are enough benefits to be gained from a particular course of action, the tendency is to ignore the accompanying costs. The person who smokes, for example, manages to ignore persistent coughing and stained fingers and teeth, just to get a nicotine lift. By ignoring the costs of smoking, and focusing on the pleasure it gives her, she allows herself to continue enjoying smoking, despite its serious health hazards.

Human beings are very good at distorting or denying the very real health costs of a particular behavior pattern—whether it is smoking, eating inappropriately, or not exercising—in order to enjoy the rewarding aspects of such detrimental health habits. Denial of the costs of bad habits or the rationalization of these behaviors often leads to procrastination in starting a change effort or loss of motivation once an effort is begun. People may put off efforts to manage their weight, or if they do try, they give up before reaching their goal. If they do reach goal, subsequent denial and rationalization will also undermine efforts to stay at goal weight.

Immediate vs. Delayed Consequences

Some of the benefits and costs associated with a behavior are immediate: When a person eats a hearty meal, she feels satisfied. When she overeats, she feels uncomfortable. Some benefits and costs are delayed: The successful dieter will eventually be able to wear a smaller size, but not for a while. If the obese person doesn't lose weight, she may some day develop diabetes or some other obesity-related health problem.

The benefits and costs that have the most powerful influence on how a person acts are those that occur immediately, at the time the person is doing something. Long-term results that come later have far less influence.

When faced with the choice of whether to eat a hot fudge sundae now and get pleasure, or pass it up and lose weight so she can wear nicer clothes later, it is much easier for the would-be dieter to decide, "I'll start tomorrow." When the alarm goes off a half hour earlier than usual to remind her to get out and jog, the pleasure of continuing to sleep now is often more compelling than the exhilaration of completed exercise an hour from now, or of better health months or years from now.

What You Can Do

Unfortunately, as you progress in changing your habits—and trying to maintain new ones—it is easy for your thoughts to turn to the benefits of not bothering to manage weight. You may have more and more memories of when you were able to eat whatever you wanted and not worry much about calories or fat in the diet. Resentment at having to make time to exercise or pass up sugary desserts can creep into your consciousness. Such thoughts and feelings will ultimately lead to a return to old habits.

To be successful in losing and managing weight, you need to keep both the benefits you expect from managing weight, and the costs you pay for not doing so, in the forefront of your thinking at all times. At the same time, you need to refute and discredit the rewards and benefits you might expect from giving up weight management efforts, and to minimize the costs of maintaining a weight management effort.

You need to "reframe" your thinking about how things were before you undertook to manage your weight. To reframe something—an event or a situation—means to change the meaning you give it. For example, instead of seeing yourself as having to *give up* certain pleasures, think of having *gained* healthier habits that serve you better. Instead of feeling deprived because you can't eat anything you want, focus on feeling good about making wise choices that demonstrate your ability to manage yourself.

If you do have a slip, resist the temptation to take this as evidence that you are a failure. Ask yourself, "What can I learn from this so that next time I'll do better?" When you start thinking about how easy it used to be (when you weren't bothering with managing weight), remind yourself that you also sometimes felt unhappy with behavior and dissatisfied with your appearance.

You need to constantly bring your focus back to what you expect to get by successfully managing weight. When you find yourself thinking that it is too much trouble, or that you want to give up, you need to immediately reframe these thoughts, and orient your thinking back to why getting to and staying at your best weight is important to you.

The *Benefits and Costs Analysis* form on page 24 is designed to help you assess the benefits and costs you expect from either managing weight or not bothering. Filling it out will help you increase and maintain your motivation.

Before completing the form, take a look at the sample on page 23 to get an idea of how to fill this out for yourself.

Instructions

In box #1, note the benefits you expect to get both now and later by undertaking and maintaining a weight management effort. Unfortunately, the benefits expected from weight management are usually the least well thought out. You need to develop persuasive but realistic ideas of the benefits you expect to receive from reducing weight. Moreover, these benefits must be important to you, regardless of what others think. If the benefits you expect for reducing weight are not powerful enough to compete successfully with the benefits for not doing so, or if they are not powerful enough to overcome the costs involved in losing weight, you must give this more thought. Your odds of long-term success will not be good unless you find more powerful reasons for wanting to lose weight.

Consider carefully what you write in box #1. Whatever you write should conform to the following three criteria:

1. **It must be *realistic*.** Can you reasonably expect to get this by managing weight?

2. **It must be *relevant* to you.** Is it what you really value, or is it what someone else thinks is important? If it's not important to you, it's not relevant.

3. **It must be *powerful* enough** to compete with the benefits of not losing weight, powerful enough to outweigh the costs of trying to manage weight.

In completing this analysis, one woman wrote that the benefits she expected to get from managing weight were to be able to wear a size nine dress and get more compliments. The therapist asked if she presently got compliments from her husband and people she cared about. The woman replied that she did. The therapist then asked if her husband and friends particularly cared if she wore a size nine or a size 16. The woman conceded they probably didn't.

"Is wearing a size nine dress going to be powerful enough to carry you through the tough times when you don't feel like exercising or do feel like eating inappropriately?" inquired the therapist.

"I guess not," replied the woman.

"Then you need to rethink your reasons for wanting to lose weight. Try to develop some really powerful but realistic ideas about what being slimmer will do for you. Don't start weight reduction efforts until you do."

Benefits and Costs Analysis   sample

#1 Benefits of Losing Weight?
What do you expect to get, now or later, that you want? What do you get to avoid that would be unpleasant?

— feel better physically
—able to put on pantyhose
     without getting out of breath
—wear pretty clothes
—like myself more

#3 Costs Involved in Losing Weight?
What do you have to do or give up that you don't want to do or give up? What do you have to do that you would rather not do?

—give up junk food
—cut down on alcohol
—make time for exercise

#2 Benefits of Not Losing Weight?
What do you get to do that you enjoy doing? What do you avoid having to do?

—don't have to deal with men
—don't risk getting hurt
—eat & drink what I want
—control is unnecessary
—don't have to exercise

#4 Costs of Not Losing Weight?
What unpleasant or undesirable things are you likely to get now or in the future? What are you likely to lose?

—poor health
—feeling fat
—feeling bad about mysellf
—lack of a relationship
—hard to get around; tired, out of breath

Benefits and Costs Analysis

#1 Benefits of Losing Weight?

What do you expect to get, now or later, that you want? What do you get to avoid that would be unpleasant?

#3 Costs Involved in Losing Weight?

What do you have to do or give up that you don't want to do or give up? What do you have to do that you would rather not do?

#2 Benefits of Not Losing Weight?

What do you get to do that you enjoy doing? What do you avoid having to do?

#4 Costs of Not Losing Weight?

What unpleasant or undesirable things are you likely to get now or in the future? What are you likely to lose?

In box #2, indicate the benefits you expect to get now and later by not bothering to manage weight. These might sound like, "not having to make an effort to exercise," "being able to enjoy my wine and cheese after work," "continuing to snack on candy bars," and so forth. These are the sorts of things you get to enjoy right now when you are not trying to control weight, and these are the things that are most likely to come to mind when you are paying the costs of losing weight.

In box #3, state the costs you expect to pay now and later by undertaking weight reduction efforts. In the enthusiasm of a fresh effort at losing weight, you may be tempted to ignore or minimize these. Don't. Acknowledge them now and make an informed decision to pay these costs. It is important to recognize and acknowledge them in the beginning, so that they will not come as a surprise later. (When you find yourself thinking about them in the future, you will want to discount and minimize them as much as possible, and to turn your attention back to what you have noted in boxes #1 and #4.)

Finally, in box #4, write the costs you now pay and may pay in the future by not managing weight. Once your change effort is underway, your natural tendency will be to deny or minimize the costs you pay for not losing weight. By putting them down now, it will be harder to dismiss them later. Be honest with yourself here; it will be important to you later.

When a person is anticipating beginning a weight management program, the boxes that tend to exert the most influence on behavior are boxes #1 and #4—the benefits of losing weight and the costs of not losing weight. As a result, the person feels motivated to get going. On the other hand, people who focus on boxes #2 and #3—the benefits of not changing and the costs of managing weight—find it hard to start a weight management effort or to stay with one.

These "de-motivation" boxes are shaded on your form as a reminder that to be successful in managing weight, you must minimize such ideas as much as possible. If you find your thoughts focusing on the ideas in the shaded boxes, reorient your thinking to the ideas in the unshaded "motivation" boxes—box #1 (the benefits you expect to get from changing) and box #4 (the costs you will pay for not changing). By staying focused on these, you can motivate yourself to undertake a weight reduction effort and stick with it.

Periodically you should go back and review your *Benefits and Costs Analysis* form. As you progress in your weight management efforts, you may find new reasons to continue with your effort, or you may need to acknowledge and accept some costs you hadn't recognized previously. You should plan to do this regularly. Use this analysis form to keep your commitment clear and your motivation on track. It also helps to post this form some place where you will see it frequently—perhaps on the refrigerator door.

Summary

Life is about trade-offs. Every decision, every action leads to consequences, some of which are desirable, others undesirable. So too is deciding to undertake a weight management effort. Most people focus only on the challenge of losing weight, assuming that once they get to goal weight everything will be fine. Rarely is it considered that being at goal weight has it's down side as well.

There are pros and cons to the decision to lose and maintain a lower body weight. It is important to consider in advance, the benefits and costs of this decision, so that you will be better prepared for the challenges of keeping off the weight once you've lost it.

References

1.   O'Connell, D., & Velicer, W.F. (1989). A decisional balance measure and the stages of change model for weight loss. *International Journal of the Addictions, 23,* 729–750.

Chapter 3

Learning to "Think Smart"

BETTY LAUGHED at the suggestion she try and get the support and cooperation of her family and friends in her weight management efforts.

"I have to entertain my husband's clients, and they expect to be served fancy meals.

"I couldn't ask my family and friends to treat me in a special way; it's not fair to put my problem on them. Besides, I should be able to handle this myself."

Pat kept putting off the new clothes she needed for work, telling herself that she should lose some weight first. She bought every diet book that was published, but didn't read them. She joined a weight reduction program several times, but never lost a pound. Her job took up most of her energy, and it was difficult to fit dieting or exercise into her schedule. As her weight crept steadily upward, she found herself with less and less energy and less and less confidence in being able to do anything about her weight.

Marie decided she was going to lose weight by eating only one meal a day. She succeeded with this plan for several days, until she visited her daughter who had just baked some fresh cookies. Marie ate one, and that was the end of her diet. She went right back to eating as she had before, and she felt depressed and angry with herself for having done so badly.

Betty, Pat, and Marie are all caught in *thinking traps*—ways of thinking that lead to procrastination, decreased motivation, failures, and painful emotions. Thinking traps have been called "distorted thinking"[1] or "cognitive distortions"[2] by some psychologists. They are simply ways of thinking that cause a person to deny or distort information, and lead to ineffective action or action that produces an undesired result. Like the "bugs" in a computer program, thinking traps make it difficult for a person to get what she wants.

Some thinking traps are created by the way you process the information of your senses in order to make sense out of what happens to you, and others are products of the beliefs you hold. Using the computer metaphor again, some errors in thinking are because of the glitches in the software program you use—that is, what goes into processing the information—and other errors come from your data base—your beliefs.

In order to avoid thinking traps, you need to better understand how you think, how beliefs affect action, and how faulty thinking is involved. Then you can take the steps necessary to start "thinking smart."

The Process of Thinking

You think in both words and pictures. When you talk to yourself, you are thinking "verbally," or thinking in words. When you visualize something in your mind's eye, or "hear" a melody in your memory, or "smell" a smell that isn't there any more, you are thinking in pictures or images.

When you think in pictures and images, you may also feel emotions that go with the pictures and images. "Verbal" thinking may accompany "picture" thinking, and both kinds of thinking can go on at once.

Different parts of the brain are responsible for different kinds of thinking.[3] The left half of the brain is primarily in charge of thinking in words. It is involved in logical, rational and verbal thinking. The right half of the brain thinks mostly in pictures and images, and perhaps emotions. This thinking is nonrational (but not irrational), nonlinear, and nonverbal.

Right-brain thinking is "picture" thinking. With this kind of thinking you can know something but not be able to explain how it is that you know it. If you are like most people, you are probably more aware of your verbal or left-brain thinking than you are of your picture or right-brain thinking.

Aspects of Thinking

Level of Consciousness

Some thinking is on a conscious level—that is, you are aware of what you are thinking—and some is at a preconscious or subconscious level. In the latter case, thinking is said to be "out of awareness." Certain techniques can be used to bring some out-of-awareness thinking into consciousness. Some of these techniques include free association, sentence completions, guided imagery, and hypnosis.

Even conscious thinking can be brought into sharper focus, through writing in a journal or keeping a record of thoughts associated with certain behaviors. This is exactly what you do when you write down what you eat and any associated thoughts you may be having at the time. By keeping such a record, you develop greater awareness of the thoughts and feelings that are associated with your eating behavior, and you may become aware of things that weren't readily available to consciousness before.

Awareness

Awareness influences behavior by focusing conscious attention on certain information.* Self-awareness is a particular kind of awareness, and is important for successful weight management. A study of both obese and normal weight people had some subjects eat in front of a mirror while other subjects did not have a mirror. Those who ate in front of the mirror ate less than those without the mirror. Awareness of eating behavior influences how people eat.

Developing greater awareness is the first step to taking charge of your thinking. Because much of the way you think is learned, you have more control over your thinking than you may realize—and by extension, you have more control over your behavior, because, as you will see, thinking guides behavior.

Selective Attention

At all times you are surrounded by more information from your environment than you can possibly absorb. You must choose what to notice and what to ignore.

Very early in your development, your culture and the people you are close to, teach you what to notice and what distinctions to make. If you are an Eskimo, for example, you can distinguish between many different kinds of snow. An avid skier may distinguish at least three kinds of snow (powder, packed, corn snow), but if you are a native Floridian still living in Florida, you probably think there is only one kind of snow. What you notice and the distinctions you make are learned in part from your culture.

Store of Information

As you developed from infancy to adulthood, you learned from your parents and from your environment what was important to pay attention to and what was not. You also adopted certain ideas about how things are, about right and wrong, about how things should and shouldn't be, and about what is important and what isn't so important. All along the way you made decisions about yourself, about other people, and about your world that have impact on the way you think today. All of this information is stored in memory and is analogous to the data base a computer draws upon to process information.

---

* Some scientists argue that awareness can go on outside of consciousness too, as in subliminal perception. While this may be true, what is of concern here is conscious awareness.

Giving Meaning

Once something has entered your awareness and you attend to it, the next step is to decide what it means to you and what, if anything, you need to do. As a result of what you decide about the event, you are also likely to experience some emotions or feelings.

When Marie broke her diet by eating one of her daughter's cookies, she became angry with herself and decided that this meant she was too weak-willed to manage her weight. As a result of the meaning she gave to eating the cookie, she gave up her dieting efforts.

That meaning was quite arbitrary, however. She might just as well have decided that eating one cookie wasn't necessarily evidence of a personal failing. She could have taken it instead as a signal to reevaluate the way she was trying to lose weight and perhaps to choose a more appropriate method.

The meaning you give to a particular event will depend in part on your beliefs, values, expectations, past experiences, and other inputs you use for the thinking process. The degree to which you are caught in certain "thinking traps" associated with these inputs will affect the meaning you give to what happens around you.

The process of giving meaning to some thing or event usually leads to some kind of behavior. Sometimes you simply store the meaning in your memory, along with any emotions you feel at the time. Later, you may recall the memory, reexperience the emotion, and attempt to cope in some way. Other times, you react directly to the meaning you have placed on a thing or event and the emotion you feel.

When Marie broke her diet, she decided this meant she couldn't control her eating, so she went back to inappropriate eating behavior. For some people, a small indiscretion such as this might lead to an eating binge. When you experience an event that you perceive as stressful, you may find that you reach for something to eat, or drink, or smoke, in order to feel better—that is, to cope with the stress. You then notice how you acted, and this becomes additional information that influences how you perceive the event and the decisions you make about yourself and your ability to cope.

Beliefs: Filters for Viewing the World

Your beliefs are like eye glasses that you look through to see and understand the world, except that instead of making your vision more clear, these glasses can distort. Your beliefs color how you see things. For example, if you believe in democracy, you value personal freedom, and are more likely to allow different points of view to be expressed. If you believe in communism, however, you value the state above the person, and are less likely to tolerate conflicting ideas.

If you believe that obesity results from a weak will and indulgent overeating, you are likely to regard an obese person with disgust. If you realize that obesity is a complex problem that involves physiological, psychological, cultural, and social variables, and is not merely the result of self-indulgence, you are more likely to feel compassion for an obese person. Depending on the beliefs you hold, you will see things a particular way and act accordingly.

Obese Beliefs

Shulabith Kreitler and Abigail Chemerinski have studied how four types of beliefs concerning 20 different themes distinguish between those who have weight problems and those who don't.[4] According to these researchers, the obese tend more to have a particular way of interpreting their weight problems.

The obese tend to reject notions of self-control, and avoid having to place limitations on themselves. They also reject the possibility of change, and tend to avoid the open expression of emotions, especially hostile ones.

In addition, the obese are overly concerned about interpersonal relations, especially issues related to dependence, vulnerability, and differences between themselves and others. They strive for achievement, but work hard to avoid confronting difficult issues. Although they may be obsessively concerned with how to lose or control weight, they tend to be ineffective in their efforts and react to failure with guilt.

The researchers concluded that, unless such beliefs are changed, there is little hope that weight management can be effective.

Irrational Beliefs

Albert Ellis is a psychologist who was among the first to examine how beliefs and the way you think influence behavior and your emotional experience.[5] He gives twelve "irrational ideas" that he believes contribute to poor thinking.

Examine the following list based on Ellis' ideas, and see if any of these are ideas or beliefs that you hold. If so, work on replacing them with the more rational alternative suggested.

These irrational ideas are thinking traps that not only lead to painful emotions, but also make it more difficult to manage weight effectively. Holding onto these beliefs and applying them inflexibly produces many problems.

Irrational Ideas and *Rational Alternatives*

1. The idea that it is a dire necessity for me to be loved and respected by everyone for everything I do,

INSTEAD OF concentrating on setting my own standards, winning my own self-respect, regarding approval from others as my preference rather than a necessity, and on loving rather than being loved.

2. The idea that I should be thoroughly competent, intelligent, and achieving in all possible respects, setting high standards and not being satisfied with a mediocre achievement,

INSTEAD OF doing my best, striving to be excellent but not perfect, and accepting my own human limitations and specific fallibilities.

3. The idea that it is horrible and awful when things are not the way I want them to be,

INSTEAD OF striving to change or control those conditions that can be changed, and when necessary, accepting the way things are.

4. The idea that I need someone stronger or greater than myself on which to rely,

INSTEAD OF taking risks and acting independently.

5. The idea that because something strongly affected me in the past, this must continue to affect me, or because things turned out badly before, they are likely to again,

INSTEAD OF letting go of past experiences, refusing to allow them to have power over me, and learning from these past experiences.

6. The idea that I must be in control at all times,

INSTEAD OF realizing that it is impossible to always be in control and learning to relax and even enjoy new challenges and situations.

Irrational Ideas *and* *Rational Alternatives*

7. The idea that it is easier to avoid than to face up to burdens, life difficulties, or personal responsibiiities,

INSTEAD OF realizing that putting off facing problems only makes them worse to deal with in the long-run, and by facing up to and handling a problem now I will feel better sooner.

8. The idea that I can be happy if I'm left alone or not involved in outside pursuits,

INSTEAD OF realizing that happines comes from being absorbed in creative pursuits and from devoting myself to people and projects outside myself.

9. The idea that some things people do are awful or wicked, and that those who do these things should be severely punished,

INSTEAD OF realizing that the way in which people behave is always the result of their judgment about what is best or appropriate for them, even though their acts may in fact be stupid, neurotic, or criminal, and that they should be helped to change if possible, and failing that, prevented from committing such acts again.

10. The idea that I should be upset about, or even retreat from, something that might be fearsome or dangerous,

INSTEAD OF realizing it is better to face up frankly to it and cope with it, or else accept the inevitable in relative calm.

11. The idea that my suffering and misery are caused be other people and events,

INSTEAD OF realizing that my experience of suffering and misery is caused by the *view* I take of the conditions, and I would be better off looking for ways to change things.

12. The idea that I can't help how I feel or that my emotions are in charge of me,

INSTEAD OF realizing that I have enormous control over my emotions, if only I learn to "think smart" and use appropriate techniques for controlling emotional arousal.

Common Thinking Traps
Rigid Rules

Another way to think about beliefs is to think of them as "rules." Your system of beliefs is like having a rule book that you carry around in your head—it tells you how things are or how they are supposed to be.

Unfortunately, when you apply rigid rules and lack flexibility in your thinking, you are caught in yet another thinking trap. You insist that your rules be followed and forget that other people don't always have the same rule book you have; they don't necessarily share your beliefs.

The overuse of certain words usually signals that you have fallen into this trap: "should," "shouldn't," "ought," "oughtn't," "must," "must not." If you hold rigidly to your beliefs, and refuse to make room for differences in beliefs, or at least to acknowledge that others may have another point of view, the stage is set for both emotional and interpersonal difficulty.

Betty believed that she ought to be able to manage her weight without putting a burden on others. Early on she had learned from her father that "you should always stand on your own two feet." Independence was something she held dear.

But by clinging rigidly to this notion, Betty failed to notice that by always maintaining that she didn't need anyone's help, her family felt closed out and not wanted by her. She gained some satisfaction by asserting her independence, but by trying to go it alone with weight management, she also felt frustrated, angry, and alone.

Rigidly applying beliefs acquired at an earlier time, or acting on beliefs which may now be inappropriate, is a thinking trap—one that can be avoided by being willing to take a fresh look at the long-held beliefs, and if necessary, to change them.

Filtering and Discounting

Filtering is a thinking trap that involves a kind of selective attention. When you fall into it, you notice only certain things and ignore other information. It causes you to miss data you need in order to cope more effectively and to take control of your behavior. For example, you may notice all of your faults, what you did wrong, and how you failed, but at the same time filter out your good points, what you did right, and whatever successes you may have had.

The filtering trap catches many dieters. Like them, you, too, may be able to recite examples of how you failed, and reasons why you don't have what it takes to succeed with weight management. But you don't pay much attention to the many times you have made healthy food choices, managed your behavior well, or achieved other small successes.

Giving credit where credit is due, when it comes to your eating behavior, doesn't happen. You only pay attention to what the scale says, and filter out all other information that would indicate you are succeeding in your weight management efforts. You may be like Janet.

Every week Janet came to her weight management class, and before even getting on the scale, she would enumerate all of her failings over the past week. She ate a cookie on Tuesday, and then on Wednesday she didn't exercise, and on Thursday she had a glass of wine that she shouldn't have had, and so on.

When questioned about her behavior in between these "failings," she would admit hesitantly, "Well, yes, I did exercise five days this week, and yes, I weighed and measured my food every day, but . . . ," and she would protest that she hadn't lost enough weight to really count these as successes.

When positive information did get past Janet's filters, as when the scale showed that indeed she had lost weight, Janet fell into yet another thinking trap—discounting the evidence of her success. She de-emphasized the importance of having lost weight and focused more on her perceived short-comings during the week.

This distorted view of her behavior and her success kept her from seeing the bigger picture. By focusing on what she perceived as failures, she created feelings of upset, anxiety, and depression that undermined her motivation and made her experience of weight management, and indeed life, very painful.

To overcome the traps of filtering and discounting, Janet needed to change her way of thinking. She had to stop blocking out important information and start paying attention to evidence of her success as well as of her short-comings. She had to learn to notice things she had dismissed before—her own accomplishments. Once having noticed them, she needed to give herself full credit. By falling into the traps of filtering and discounting, Janet blocked out important information by choosing to notice some things and not others, and she minimized her accomplishments.

Labeling

Rebecca engaged in a different kind of faulty thinking. The thinking trap that caught her was labeling. No sooner did Rebecca meet someone than she made a judgment about them that in many cases kept her from taking seriously any information that did not confirm her original judgment. When Rebecca moved to a small, academic community from an artistic section of a large city, she decided that the people in her neighborhood were too "linear," and she just couldn't relate to them. She missed her old friends, and made few efforts to make new ones. Having labeled the people around her in a negative way, she closed off the opportunity to learn more about them, and perhaps come to like some. Feeling isolated and lonely, she ate herself into a weight problem.

Perfectionism

As a child, Marie had always gotten love and approval for outstanding performance, so she learned early to set high goals for herself. Her self-esteem depended on not making mistakes, and avoiding failure. She was caught in the trap of perfectionism.

She set high standards, and would not tolerate the slightest deviation. For her, an average performance was less than satisfying; she wanted to be perfect in what she did. Marie's house was always neat as a pin, and she never had a hair out of place. So when she wasn't perfect in following her diet, she regarded it as a complete failure. No matter that the diet she chose was inappropriate at best; she regarded her failure as a shameful display of weakness. The accompanying self-criticism produced painful feelings of frustration and anger.

The trap of perfectionism, which is also known as "polarized thinking" or "all-or-nothing thinking," involves seeing things in stark contrasts—good or bad, black or white, all or none, perfection or failure. There is little or no room for middle ground. To get out of the trap of perfectionism you must develop a different point of view, one that allows room for being human.

Making a list of the advantages and disadvantages of attempting to be perfect will usually demonstrate that being a perfectionist is not to your advantage. This can provide the motivation to work toward giving up being a perfectionist. Keeping a daily written record of self-critical thoughts helps increase awareness, and allows you to substitute thoughts that are more self-accepting. It is better to strive for "excellence"—doing or being the best that you can be at the time—rather than to strive for perfection, which involves trying to be in control at all times. Being totally in control at all times is impossible.

Exaggerated Sense of Control

Beliefs about how much control you have affect the meaning you give to things and events. Some people generally assume they have a great deal of control over events and outcomes of importance, while others tend to think that things turn out the way they do, not because of their influence, but because of luck, chance, fate, or the influence of others. In fact, how much control you have depends a lot on the situation you are in, as well as on how you tend to think about your ability to control.

Marie believed that what happened to her was almost completely within her control. As a result, she blamed herself for being weak-willed and eating the cookie. It did not occur to her that by eating only one meal a day, her willpower was seriously jeopardized by hunger and fatigue, and all it took to undo her resolve was for her daughter to urge her to just taste one cookie. The situation was working against Marie, and she had set it up that way! She blamed her willpower instead of her "skillpower."

The problem was not a flaw in her character, but a flaw in her approach to weight management. It is not possible for anyone to be completely in control of everything that happens. Rather, it is important to learn to control what is within one's realm of influence, and to let the rest take care of itself.

This is especially true for people who think they are responsible for the pain and happiness of others around them. Rose Mary put her own needs last, after the needs of her children and her spouse. She thought she was responsible not only for their happiness and comfort, but for the feelings of her parents, her siblings, her friends, and even her neighbors.

This exaggerated sense of control was evident in Rose Mary's chauffeur-ing of her adolescent children to their various activities, picking up after them and doing all the household tasks, catering to her husband's every need at night, but never having any time for herself. Rose Mary's time and energy were focused almost entirely on others, but no one had much concern for her needs. The best she seemed able to do for herself was to stuff down a couple of doughnuts in between chauffeur trips, or to grab a bowl of ice cream late at night after everyone had gone to bed. Unfortunately, it is something of an axiom that other people's needs will expand to fill the time and space you have available to take care of them.

Taking on too much responsibility for others' pain and happiness can cause you to feel like a martyr. You may create this situation because you are looking for a "hidden bargain"—you hope that all your sacrifice and self-denial will pay off some day, as if someone were keeping score. What you as the martyr don't realize is that those who are benefiting from your sacrificing are most likely taking it all for granted, and assuming that you like to make such sacrifices. When your just reward doesn't come, you are likely to feel resentful and complain that others aren't being "fair." The fallacy of fairness is yet another thinking trap.

Fallacy of Fairness

Fairness is something you learned very early, when you were asked to share your toys with another child. Teaching children to play fair helps them to learn to interact more productively with others, and is a value that could make adult interaction more satisfying; but the fact is that not everyone plays fair.

In life things happen that don't seem to be fair or just. Holding blindly to the idea that things should be fair can cause emotional upset. As a result, you may come to feel victimized or as if you have little or no control over what happens.

Minimized Sense of Control

People who do not feel they have much control over how things turn out are in the trap of being a victim. They don't take action, or when they do, it is only half-hearted, because they don't believe they have much power to influence the outcome. Because of a minimized sense of control, they often blame others or events outside themselves for what happens.

The woman who pleads that she just couldn't stop herself from eating the candy because her boss gave her a box of chocolates for her birthday, is taking a victim position. In fact, she could have anticipated this gift and suggested a better alternative, or she could simply thank her boss for the gift and immediately give the candy away to her co-workers.

The way to stop being a victim and to begin to develop a more realistic sense of control is to learn that you contribute toward the way things turn out. That is, while other factors may also be involved, you make decisions, take action, or fail to take action, and this helps to make things turn out as they do. By arbitrarily assuming that you had something to do with the way things turn out (whether or not you actually do), you are in a better position to see what corrective action can be taken in the future, so that you can exercise appropriate control.

How much control you see yourself as having can change as the situation changes. Focusing on successes in making small changes in behavior, rather than focusing just on what the scale indicates, can increase the sense of control and self-confidence you feel.

Generally, gaining a better sense of being in control of your behavior and your weight is a positive experience—one that contributes to success. Sometimes, however, the possibility of taking control can be stress-inducing. There are those who don't want to have control.

Right / Wrong Thinking

Anna developed a weight problem as a child, and as a result of it, she succeeded in getting the major share of her parents' attention, which included being taken to various doctors to find a solution to her problem and being given gifts to make her feel better. She was successful in getting far more attention from her parents than either her brother and sister.

Later, Anna lost weight and married. Shortly afterwards, she regained the weight and her husband unwittingly started treating Anna just as her parents had—bringing her gifts and giving her lots of attention for her "problem."

Finally, at the insistence of her husband, she joined a weight control program sponsored by a very prestigious university. She was very upset at the prospect of trying to lose weight, and stated that she regarded this as her last chance. During the course of the program, she gained ten pounds.

Being in control of her own behavior and having personal influence over her weight problem ran counter to the pattern of dependence and attention seeking that she had developed early in her life. Furthermore, if she indeed lost weight, she would likely cease to be the center of attention in her family.

Anna never did lose weight in the program and eventually dropped out. From her point of view, she had tried and failed, and this demonstrated that she could not take control of her problem. Anna was very invested in being right, and in confirming that she was not responsible for her weight problem. By doing so, she reaped certain benefits that in fact worked to maintain that weight problem.

Right/wrong thinking is a trap that catches many people. As a youngster you learned that it is better to be right than to be wrong. Being wrong usually brought some kind of punishment, whereas being right avoided it. So you did whatever it took to be right, even if that meant distorting the truth so that you appeared to be right when you weren't.

When you are invested in being right, you feel a need to constantly prove that your opinions and actions are correct. Being wrong is unthinkable. You insist on your point of view, even if it means shouting down the other person, coercing him or her to accept your position, or secretly holding onto your viewpoint while seeming to accept another's.

You can reduce your tendency toward right/wrong thinking by working on listening with an open mind to the other person's point of view and entertaining the notion that she may be right. Try to find a way to accommodate both your opinion and the other person's opinion so that you can both be right.

Betty did this when she stopped insisting on her notions about what constitutes a good hostess and was willing to let go of her assumptions about what guests wanted. As a result, she was able to hear the point of view advanced by her weight management instructor. She finally agreed that while some guests may expect special efforts in their behalf, that doesn't necessarily translate into high-fat/high-calorie meals. Guests can feel well treated when served healthier alternatives.

Even when the other person is right and you are wrong, this need not lead to a loss of self-esteem. For some people, being right is so important that their sense of self-esteem is threatened by seeming to be wrong. At this point they don't simply believe that being right is better than being wrong; they have made being right an important value that colors their thinking. Unfortunately, placing a high value on being right can make this thinking trap even harder to escape from. When values are involved in giving meaning to things and events, there is often less flexibility in thinking.

Taking Things Personally

Sometimes you may erroneously interpret other people's behavior. Virginia was having lunch with a large group of people, when one person at the table made a comment as another, very overweight person passed by: "How can people let themselves go like that?" Virginia, who was herself considerably overweight, interpreted the remark to be actually meant for her. She had fallen into the thinking trap of personalization—taking things personally.

The person who takes things personally tends to secretly have self-doubts about her own worth. As a result, she expects that others also don't value her very highly. Their remarks and behavior are regarded with suspicion, and she is ever alert for confirmation that they devalue her. When such confirmation seems to come (and it seems to come frequently), she reacts with hurt feelings, indignation, and withdrawal.

If you tend to take things personally, feeling that other people are putting you down or mistreating you on purpose, examine your beliefs about yourself. Low self-esteem and self-critical beliefs create the expectation that others mean to hurt you. In most cases, this is not true. The tendency to take things personally also arises from the belief that it is a dire necessity for you to be loved and respected by everyone. You need to challenge and change irrational beliefs that prompt you to take things personally.

Even if an unkind remark or act is meant for you, you don't have to take it personally. To preserve your self-esteem, you must learn how to hear and use criticism, but not let it hurt you.

Try to keep in mind that someone who is intentionally being unkind is usually hurting inside in some way. Their meanness is an attempt to deal with their own unhappiness. Or they may simply lack sufficient sensitivity to their fellow humans, perhaps having never learned to be sensitive to others, or having themselves been treated insensitively. In the face of nastiness from others, first try to see that it is really their problem, not yours.

In addition to hearing upsetting remarks as more of a statement about the speaker than about you, there is a trick you can use to protect yourself. You can protect yourself in such a situation by imagining that there is an invisible shield that surrounds you and protects you from hurting remarks or acts. Just mentally pull up your shield whenever you need it and pretend that the nasty remarks bounce off.

Over-Generalizing

Sometimes you may decide what something means based on one, seemingly relevant piece of evidence, the importance of which is then exaggerated. Deciding that you can't lose weight because you tried once and didn't succeed—and then acting as if there were overwhelming evidence for this conclusion—is an example of over-generalizing. This is similar to the trap of "jumping to a conclusion."

Jumping to a Conclusion

With no evidence, you decide what something means or, without checking it out, you decide what someone is thinking or feeling. This latter situation is also called "mind reading."

Betty fell into this trap when she concluded that her guests expected a fancy (which, for Betty, translated to "high-fat, high-calorie") meal. She jumped to this conclusion without asking her guests what they might prefer, and without even trying to prepare a meal that was appealing but not high in fat or calories. She also filtered out information that more and more people are concerned about their diet and their health and are choosing food differently. (Many restaurants are beginning to cater to this preference of their customers.) Rather, Betty decided what her guests expected and proceeded to act as if this were fact.

Dwelling on the Past

Dwelling on the past is a thinking trap that prevents you from using new information that may be more relevant to making decisions today. Past experiences can cement in beliefs that no longer work, or that cause perfectly good beliefs to be applied inappropriately.

Betty was an intelligent, powerful woman who achieved significant success in her life, partly because of a strong sense of her own competence. Much of what she has accomplished has come from being willing to strike out, be independent, and stand alone. She tried to apply this same approach to managing her weight: "I ought to be able to do this myself. I used to teach courses on how to get whatever you want by believing in yourself and going after it. So why am I unable to manage my weight?" Betty's focus on what had worked in the past, and her unwillingness to consider a different approach kept her stuck. She needed to evaluate her present situation from a fresh perspective.

Magnification / Minimization

Pat wanted to lose weight, but she also wanted to do well in her job, and it seemed to her that she couldn't do both. Her job demanded most of her time and energy, and little was left for the work of weight reduction. She was aware that her weight was causing her some health problems, and increasingly she had less energy to get through the day. She resolved the discomfort she felt in having these two, apparently conflicting values, by falling into the magnification/minimization thinking trap.

She told herself that her job achievement was more important at this point in her career, and that she couldn't afford to take the time to undertake a serious weight management effort. She rationalized that she would get around to managing her weight "one of these days." She tried to cope with her decreasing energy level by taking megadoses of vitamins and a variety of questionable health potions. Periodically she tried some new diet or quickie weight reduction scheme, only to fail each time to lose weight. Consequently, her self-esteem and her confidence that she could lose weight successfully also declined.

Because Pat valued two things, job achievement and weight reduction, that competed for her time and energy, she solved the dilemma by magnifying the importance of the job achievement, and minimizing the importance of making a serious effort to lose weight. In the meantime, years were passing and her health was beginning to suffer. As her health declined, her productivity on the job declined.

By falling into the trap of magnification/minimization, Pat ended up short-changing herself. It did not occur to her that losing excess weight could bring about an increase in energy, which could then be devoted to doing her job even better. She did not see that by adjusting priorities, at least temporarily, she might achieve both her goals.

Taking time to clarify your values can be the first step out of this thinking trap. If you find yourself procrastinating about weight management, be sure you have carefully completed the *Benefits and Costs Analysis* discussed in the previous chapter. This is in part a values clarification exercise that can help you get better focused on your values and priorities.

Failure Expectation

Feeling defeated before you even begin signals the presence of the failure expectation thinking trap. Usually the expectation of failure results from previous experiences that resulted in failure. The experience of the past is carried over to the present, and feelings of hopelessness undermine motivation to begin or continue an effort.

The more Pat observed herself not being in control of her eating behavior, the greater became her doubts about her ability to do so. Because of her continued failure, she was developing an expectation that she was not able to manage weight. With decreased self-confidence, she was less likely to begin or do well at any new weight management effort she might undertake, because she believed she couldn't succeed.

In contrast to the failure expectation that Pat developed, however, is the expectation developed by another woman. Wendy had tried every diet that came along, on two separate occasions went to a doctor for shots, and finally concluded that these approaches don't work. She didn't lose confidence in herself, just in the methods. She still believed she could succeed in managing weight with the right approach, and she kept trying. Her expectation was finally supported when she got involved in a comprehensive program involving regular exercise, nutrition education, and lifestyle changes.

Expectations are essentially decisions you make about your ability, or about the likelihood that some particular program or approach will allow you to get what you want. You create expectations based on your past experiences and your general outlook on the world, and you use expectations to make predictions about what will happen now or in the future.

You have much more control over your expectations than you may think. You can reexamine expectations based on past decisions you made, see if they are well-founded, and if necessary, change them. Calling into question expectations that keep you stuck, and making new decisions are often necessary for learning how to think smart.

Thinking and Behaving

As Shakespeare said, "Nothing is either good or bad, but thinking makes it so." The way you think influences how you feel, and thinking and feeling together influence how you act and behave. Your behavior and the results it produces provide information to you that you must make sense out of. What you decide about your actions and the consequences they bring may engender further thoughts and feelings. All of this is stored in your memory or "data bank."

Learning to "Think Smart"

Learning to identify the various kinds of thinking traps is the first step toward developing greater awareness of them. The *What's the Trap?* self-test that follows will help you assess your ability to identify various thinking traps. Match the thinking trap on the left with the thought on the right that contains the particular thinking trap in question. There is only one correct match for each thought and each thinking trap label.

As you develop greater awareness of the thinking traps that catch you, you will also be better able to get out of them, or avoid them all together. The first few times you discover yourself in one of these traps, you will probably do nothing more than notice that you are in it. For example, you may suddenly notice that you are insisting on being "right" with someone and not listening to his or her point of view. Subsequently, when you find yourself in a similar situation, you are more likely to act differently—to be open to the other person's point of view. Or you may find yourself in the process of maximizing one alternative and minimizing another, and then decide

Self-Test 3.1

What's the Trap?

Thinking Trap Label	*Thought Containing A Thinking Trap*
1. Dwelling on the Past	a. Never again will I touch another chocolate chip cookie.
2. Magnification/Minimization	b. It's not fair that others can eat whatever they want and I can't.
3. Perfectionism	c. My family expects me to cook a big meal every night; I can't ask them to change for me.
4. Fairness	d. I've tried and tried to lose weight; I guess I was just meant to be fat.
5. Right/Wrong	e. Right now I've got to focus my energies on my career; losing weight isn't as important.
6. Minimized Sense of Control	f. I got to goal weight once but gained it all back; I guess I'm just meant to be fat.
7. Filtering	g. I may be losing weight, but it's not fast enough.
8. Rigid Rules	h. My neighbor stays slim by fasting one day a week, so I'm sure fasting is okay, no matter what you say.
9. Discounting	i. My family depends on me; I have to take care of their needs first.
10. Jumping to a Conclusion	j. I can't ever be thin because I was overfed as a child and I probably have too many fat cells.
11. Over-generalization	k. You should always clean your plate.
12. Exaggerated Sense of Control	l. Everything went wrong this week; I didn't do anything right.
13. Personalization	m. She's a compulsive eater.
14. Failure Expectation	n. She really had me in mind when she said some people she knows are boring.
15. Labeling	o. I've got so much weight to lose, there's no point in even trying.

Answer Key: 1-d, 2-e, 3-a, 4-b, 5-h, 6-j, 7-i, 8-k, 9-g, 10-c, 11-f, 12-l, 13-n, 14-o, 15-m abruptly to reevaluate your thinking. As your awareness increases, you will gradually become better and better at "thinking smart."

To get better control of your thinking process and learn to "think smart," you should:

1. *Develop greater awareness.* Keep a diary of your thoughts in addition to recording what you eat.

2. *Challenge and replace beliefs and values that don't work.* Avoid being too rigid in what you believe, and be especially aware of unrealistic beliefs about perfection, control, fairness, and being right. Review the list of irrational beliefs and rational alternatives given in this chapter.

3. *Reexamine past decisions, check them against the full facts, and redecide if necessary.* Be careful that you do not over-generalize, jump to conclusions, or persist in dwelling on the past

4. *Eliminate sources of denial and distortion from your thinking.* The current chapter addresses how to identify thinking traps that distort or eliminate important information.

5. *Manage your self-talk to make it more supportive and less self-critical.* Chapter 4 is devoted to how to change self-talk.

6. *Learn how to cope better with emotions.* Chapter 7 goes into this in greater detail.

7. *Try doing things differently than you usually do and see if something changes.* Chapter 6 on *Improving Your Relationships* may be particularly helpful in this regard.

Suggested Exercises for Escaping Thinking Traps

Here are some exercises you can do to help yourself out of various thinking traps:

1.   Each morning, first thing, decide on *one* thing you can reasonably get done today that would make your day worthwhile. Be sure it is something that is really do-able today. Work to get it accomplished. If, at the end of the day, you have done it, give yourself a mental pat on the back. If it didn't get done, analyze what choices you made that undermined your resolve and what you could have done to succeed. Do this without criticizing or blaming yourself.

2.   Each evening, make a mental or written list of *all* the little successes you had over the course of the day. Include on this list any action you took, no matter how small, that advanced your progress toward some goal. Remember, the mental activity of deciding on a goal or course of action counts as a success too.

3. Make a list of all the perfectionistic beliefs or goals you hold yourself to. List the advantages and disadvantages of each of these—i.e., what you get (and don't get) by holding on to such an unrealistic goal, and what it costs you in time, energy, or emotional discomfort. Decide if the advantages of being a perfectionist outweigh the disadvantages.

4. At the end of the day, write down all the things you did today. Then rate each one from 0% to 100% according to:

1) how perfectly you did it, and

2) how satisfying it was.

Observe whether it is possible for you to get satisfaction when you aren't perfect.

5. When another person's actions are upsetting to you, pretend that he or she is a mirror, and is reflecting back to you some part of yourself that either:

1) you recognize but judge to be ugly or unacceptable,

2) refuse to see in yourself, or

3) would secretly like to express.

Decide how that person's behavior can teach you a lesson about yourself.

6. Make a list of all the things, persons, or situations you feel responsible for. Mark each item according to whether the item involves:

1) your physical safety and well-being, (Me Category)

2) someone else's physical safety and well-being, or (Them Category)

3) both yours and someone else's safety and well-being. (Both Category)

Now go back over the "both" items and allocate them to either the "me" or the "them" category. Cross off all the items in the "them" category. Work at being responsible only for the items in the "me" category. (Note: Many items that you think should be in the "me" category really belong in the "them" category. When in doubt, put them in the latter.)

7. Circle all the irrational ideas listed on pages 32–33 that apply to you. Using a separate index card for each idea, and using your own words, write down an alternative way of thinking about that idea that is more "rational." Keep this set of index cards with you. Read one each day and think about the alternative you have come up with.

Summary

Thinking traps introduce distortions and bias into your ability to make sense of the events that happen around you. Your belief system and your expectations are filters through which you view your world. Beliefs, especially "irrational" ones, are another source of bias. One of the most important factors in successful weight management is how you think—the cognitive distortions, beliefs, and expectations that introduce bias into your understanding of things. To ensure long-term success, you need to overcome these thinking traps and learn to think smarter.

References

1. McKay, M., Davis, M., & Fanning, P. (1981). *Thoughts and Feelings: The Art of Cognitive Stress Intervention*. Oakland, CA: New Harbinger Publications.

2. Burns, D.D. (1980). *Feeling Good: The New Mood Therapy*. New York: New American Library.

3. Levy, J. (1985). Right brain, left brain: Fact and fiction. *Psychology Today, 19,* 38–44.

4. Kreitler, S. & Chemerinski, A. (1988). the cognitive orientation of obesity. *International Journal of Obesity, 12,* 403–415.

5. Ellis, A., & Harper, R.A. (1975). *A New Guide to Rational Living*. Englewood Cliffs, NJ: Prentice-Hall, Inc.

Chapter 4

Using Self-Talk Effectively

HAVE YOU NOTICED that little voice inside your head that keeps talking to you? You know, the one that just said, "What little voice?" That voice is part of your thinking process. It has been called "verbal thinking," "stream of consciousness," "automatic thoughts," and "inner dialogue." Simply put, it is a part of your thinking that involves talking to yourself.

Perhaps there was a time when you misplaced your keys and found yourself saying out loud, "Now where are those keys? Let's see—did I leave them on the desk? No. Go look in the kitchen. There they are. Next time hang them on the key rack so you can find them." That's self-talk. Sometimes you do it out loud when no one is around. Most of the time it goes on inside your head.

Often your self-talk is very critical and judgmental. It is always noticing when someone else doesn't do something right: "She shouldn't insist I eat the cake she made," or, "He should know not to bring home candy when I'm trying to lose weight."

When you are excessively critical of others, you are likely to feel frustrated or angry and to show your disapproval. As a result, you foster negative reactions on the part of others. This often interferes with your relationships. Learning to be less judgmental and more accepting of others not only feels better for you, but usually improves the quality of your relationships as well.

Your self-talk also can be very critical of you. At times it may sound like a scolding parent, pointing out all your faults and commenting on your shortcomings. Your self-talk may discount your achievements or attribute your success to luck, timing, or accidents of fate.

When you are excessively self-critical or self-discounting, you make yourself feel depressed and demoralized. As a result, you may procrastinate or give up prematurely. Or you may set unrealistic goals and become a "workaholic" to try and compensate. On the other hand, when you are more self-accepting, you tend to set more flexible goals, to get the results you want, and to accept credit for your achievements. You generally feel better and more motivated.

Sometimes your self-talk allows you to be self-indulgent. It provides you with excuses and rationalizations, such as, "What the heck, I deserve a little treat. I'll start my diet tomorrow." It may take the form of self-pity: "Poor me, I have to give up everything I like." Or your self-talk may exaggerate: "Why does just looking at food make me fat when others can eat whatever they want?"

When your self-talk is indulgent or self-pitying, it keeps you stuck in bad habits. It produces procrastination or poor results. On the other hand, when you take a problem-solving approach to a problem and use instructional self-talk to remind yourself of what to do and how to stay on track, you can get through difficult situations and make progress toward your goal.

What you say to yourself can actually create or escalate emotions. By thinking catastrophizing thoughts and worrying about "what if...," you can make yourself feel upset, anxious, fearful, and even panic-stricken. How you talk to yourself can make already painful emotions worse, undermine resolve, and destroy motivation. It can make you feel bored, lonely, and unproductive.

These are examples of negative self-talk. As noted in Chapter 1, negative self-talk is any kind of thought that keeps you from getting to your goal. It undermines motivation, hinders coping behavior, and is self-defeating. Negative self-talk affects how others respond to you, how you feel, and how you act.

Although it is probably unlikely, and even undesirable that you could get rid of negative self-talk completely, it is important to decrease the amount of negative self-talk you use. When you find yourself thinking negatively, you can tell yourself to "stop," and switch to more positive thoughts.

In contrast to negative self-talk, positive self-talk is a coping thought that facilitates achievement of a goal. It demonstrates a flexible, accepting attitude toward yourself and others. Positive self-talk comments on the good news: "I exercised five times this week, and I feel just great," instead of focusing on the one time this week you skipped an exercise session. It makes even-handed evaluations, as in, "Overall it was a good week, and I'm pleased with my eating behavior," instead of, "I don't know how I lost any weight because I only exercised twice this week."

Positive self-talk also reflects a problem-solving approach; it helps you do things and keeps you on track. It reminds you of what to do and how to do it, as when it says, "Don't buy that. If it's in the house you'll eat it, so just forget it." Positive self-talk usually makes you feel better, happier, more motivated. Even so, it can be stern when necessary to get you refocused on your goal.

Self-talk affects you in all facets of your life—your career, your relationships, and your weight loss efforts. It either keeps you stuck in old behavior patterns or helps you succeed in making important changes.

Changing the balance of your self-talk from being predominantly critical, discounting, self-indulgent, emotionally upsetting, and self-defeating, to being predominantly accepting, accountable, supportive, emotionally soothing, and goal facilitating gets you unstuck, and helps you manage weight more effectively.

Self-Talk and The Golden Ratio

Self-talk has long been the object of religious, philosophical, and popular interest. Around the turn of the century, the famous psychologist, William James, wrote about the "religion of healthy mindedness" espoused by a variety of religious organizations.

This "mind cure movement" included not only Christian Scientists, but also lesser known groups such as the New Thoughters, the Don't Worry Movement, and the Gospel of Relaxation. The concept guiding the mind cure movement was that "thoughts are things," and that negative thinking is as destructive as putting poison in the body. Positive thinking was advocated as an antidote to the debilitating effects of negative self-talk.

Recasting these ideas into less theological terms, Norman Vincent Peale's *Power of Positive Thinking* represents a popular application of these ideas. Now modern day scientists such as Albert Ellis, Aaron Beck, and Donald Meichenbaum have climbed on the band wagon, publishing books on the subject for both professionals and lay public.

Among these scientists, however, a controversy has broken out about which kind of self-talk is more relevant—negative self-talk or positive self-talk. Ellis advocates focusing attention on attacking negative thoughts and eliminating them. Meichenbaum promotes increasing positive thinking, especially self-instructional self-statements. Beck advocates identifying a variety of "automatic thoughts" and making changes that seem appropriate.

Other scientists, Robert M. Schwartz and Gregory L. Garamoni, propose that the controversy can be resolved by not only taking into account both positive and negative self-talk, but also by identifying the best ratio of positive to negative. They contend that the best ratio is defined by what is called the "golden section proportion"—another term for the Golden Ratio.[2]

The Golden Ratio is actually an ancient concept known to both Eastern and Western cultures.* Simplified, the Golden Ratio is 2:1. That is, when the

---

* Technically, the Golden Ratio is defined as the ratio that obtains between two parts when the smaller (a) is to the larger part (b) as the larger part (b) is to the whole (a+b). That is, the smaller part of the ratio approximates 38%, while the larger part approximates 62%.

larger part is about twice as big as the smaller part, the larger part is referred to as the "golden number" and the whole as the Golden Ratio.

According to Schwartz and Garamoni, many examples of the Golden Ratio can be found through the centuries and into modern day. In ancient Greece, the Pythagoreans ascribed moral and mystical significance to the Golden Ratio, and architects of the Parthenon used it to structure the facade of this and other Greek temples. Aristotle spoke of the "golden mean." During the Middle Ages, it was known as the "divine proportion," and Kepler called it one of the "great treasures of geometry."

Many examples of the Golden Ratio exist in nature. For example, any two chambers of the nautilus shell exhibit the one-third, two-thirds proportion.

More recently, scientists have found that the Golden Ratio defines the most optimal ratio in the communication of information. Now scientists are even investigating this concept with regard to thinking, and the emerging evidence indicates that, indeed, the Golden Ratio holds.

Schwartz and Garamoni contend, based on their work, that the optimal ratio, which they call the "positive dialogue," consists of 62% positive self-talk, and 38% negative self-talk. A percentage of positive self-talk that is substantially higher than 62% indicates the person is engaging in "Pollyanna" thinking and is missing important information. When the amount of positive self-talk falls below 62%, thinking is progressively more negative—and progressively more maladaptive. Those whose self-talk is almost all negative are usually suffering severe depression or serious mental illness.

It appears that healthy mindedness is indeed defined by the Golden Ratio. The trick is, how to move toward it and away from unhealthy thinking. That is the focus of the rest of this chapter.

Taking Control of Self-Talk

Developing Awareness

The first step in taking control of self-talk is to develop a greater awareness of how you actually talk to yourself. A good place to begin is to keep a record of what you eat and what you are thinking when you eat. This technique, called "self-monitoring," helps you uncover the typical things you say to yourself related to eating, and can help you to see how your self-talk may be influencing your eating behavior.

Another way to "tune in" to your self-talk is to stop periodically throughout your day and inspect your thoughts. You can create reminders to do this, by placing stick-on dots from the stationery store on places you typically glance at throughout the day.

For example, put a dot on your wrist watch, or your mirror, or the speedometer of your car. When you see a dot, you are reminded to stop for a moment and inspect your self-talk. If you find yourself being critical, discounting yourself, making excuses, or being negative, take a moment to replace that self-talk with accepting, accountable, supportive, and encouraging thoughts.

The *Assessing Your Negative Self-Talk* self-test on pages 53–55 is another tool to help you increase your self-talk awareness. The statements given in this self-test capture the essence of much negative self-talk that undermines weight management efforts. Rate yourself from "1," (Never or rarely think this way), to "10," (Always or frequently think this way) on each item. The exact words may not be what you say to yourself, but the general idea conveyed in the statement may be familiar to you.

When you have completed the test, underline or mark those statements on which you rated yourself a six or higher. These indicate the negative self-talk you need to change. Compare the negative self-talk you typically use with the suggested counterarguments given for those statements in the section below on *Reducing Your Negative Self-Talk*.

Reducing Your Negative Self-Talk

If you find that your self-talk, your little voice, is highly critical and judgmental, or self-discounting, or self-indulgent, or emotionally upsetting, or causes you to act in ways counterproductive to weight management, you need to retrain the way you are thinking. You need to teach your little voice to be more objective and supportive—like a coach is for a team.

When you allow your self-talk to be negative, you allow it to sabotage you, to rob you of motivation, and to enmesh you in painful emotions. Retraining your little voice so that it is less of a saboteur and more of a coach is the key.

Consider what a good coach does. The job of a coach is to provide guidance, inspiration, and praise. A coach is not a "Pollyanna" that only says nice things or affirms good intentions. A coach tells the truth—objectively—without belittling or demeaning. A coach provides direction and support and calls attention to reality. A coach inspires, praises, and gives credit. Sometimes a coach kicks a little butt—but in a supportive way.

Compare the examples of negative self-talk on pages 56–62 that can sabotage you, with the kind of supportive and encouraging statements that a coach might say. Take at look the examples of negative self-talk given in the column labeled "The Saboteur Speaking." Some of these may sound familiar to you, like something you have said or thought to yourself. Pay special attention to the ones that ring true for you. Then read the counterarguments

(text continues on page 63)

Self-Test 4.1

Assessing Your Negative Self-Talk

	Never or rarely think this way.								Always or frequently think this way.	

1. I'll start tomorrow. 1 2 3 4 5 6 7 8 9 10

2. There's no use in trying. 1 2 3 4 5 6 7 8 9 10

3. Never again will I touch a _____. (particular food) 1 2 3 4 5 6 7 8 9 10

4. From now on I'm not going to _____. (do some action) 1 2 3 4 5 6 7 8 9 10

5. I'm going to lose _____ pounds. (number) 1 2 3 4 5 6 7 8 9 10

6. I'm going to _____ every day. (take some action) 1 2 3 4 5 6 7 8 9 10

7. I've got so much weight to lose that there's no point in even trying. 1 2 3 4 5 6 7 8 9 10

8. I've tried before and not succeeded, so why should things be different now? 1 2 3 4 5 6 7 8 9 10

9. I'm not losing weight; there must be something wrong with me. 1 2 3 4 5 6 7 8 9 10

10. Losing just a little weight each week is discouraging. (OR: I'm not losing weight fast enough.) 1 2 3 4 5 6 7 8 9 10

11. I'm gaining weight; I may as well quit. 1 2 3 4 5 6 7 8 9 10

12. No one else really cares, what's the use trying. 1 2 3 4 5 6 7 8 9 10

13. Other people are making this more difficult for me; maybe I should give up. 1 2 3 4 5 6 7 8 9 10

14. Poor me, I have to give up almost everything I like. 1 2 3 4 5 6 7 8 9 10

15. It's not fair that others can eat what they want and I can't. 1 2 3 4 5 6 7 8 9 10

16. Others get bored by people who are preoccupied with their weight; I'm not fun to be around when I'm dieting. 1 2 3 4 5 6 7 8 9 10

17. It's not right to make others suffer because I want to lose weight. 1 2 3 4 5 6 7 8 9 10

18. I can't ask my children and my family to change their way of eating for me. 1 2 3 4 5 6 7 8 9 10

(continued)

Self-Test 4.1

Assessing Your Negative Self-Talk (continued)

	Never or rarely think this way.								Always or frequently think this way.	
19. If I don't lose weight, my family and friends will be unhappy.	1	2	3	4	5	6	7	8	9	10
20. If I don't lose weight before _____ _____, it will be terrible. (some event)	1	2	3	4	5	6	7	8	9	10
21. What if I slip and regain weight; I couldn't stand it.	1	2	3	4	5	6	7	8	9	10
22. What if I've got too many fat cells and I'm just "naturally" fat?	1	2	3	4	5	6	7	8	9	10
23. What if this program doesn't work?	1	2	3	4	5	6	7	8	9	10
24. What if I don't have enough willpower?	1	2	3	4	5	6	7	8	9	10
25. If I don't lose weight, he (she) won't love me anymore.	1	2	3	4	5	6	7	8	9	10
26. Anyone as fat as I am doesn't deserve to feel good about herself.	1	2	3	4	5	6	7	8	9	10
27. No one could like anyone as fat as I am.	1	2	3	4	5	6	7	8	9	10
28. Life will be better when I lose this weight.	1	2	3	4	5	6	7	8	9	10
29. If I hate myself enough, maybe I'll change.	1	2	3	4	5	6	7	8	9	10
30. Gee, wouldn't that taste good.	1	2	3	4	5	6	7	8	9	10
31. I can't handle that particular food; maybe I'm addicted to it.	1	2	3	4	5	6	7	8	9	10
32. It smells (looks) so good—I just can't resist it.	1	2	3	4	5	6	7	8	9	10
33. I'm so hungry; I've got to eat.	1	2	3	4	5	6	7	8	9	10
34. I just can't stop thinking about eating.	1	2	3	4	5	6	7	8	9	10
35. I just can't resist eating; I guess I'm just a compulsive eater.	1	2	3	4	5	6	7	8	9	10
36. It tasted so good; I'd really like to have more.	1	2	3	4	5	6	7	8	9	10

Self-Test 4.1

Assessing Your Negative Self-Talk (continued)

	Never or rarely think this way.								Always or frequently think this way.	
37. If it weren't for my _____ I could lose weight. (job, kids, etc.)	1	2	3	4	5	6	7	8	9	10
38. He (or she) keeps bringing me candy (or other tempting food), so I can't lose weight.	1	2	3	4	5	6	7	8	9	10
39. She (or he) insists that I eat.	1	2	3	4	5	6	7	8	9	10
40. She (or he) would feel offended if I didn't eat.	1	2	3	4	5	6	7	8	9	10
41. With my schedule it's impossible to eat right.	1	2	3	4	5	6	7	8	9	10
42. There's too much stress in my life for me to handle managing weight.	1	2	3	4	5	6	7	8	9	10
43. I deserve a little treat now and then.	1	2	3	4	5	6	7	8	9	10
44. I paid for it; I'm going to eat it.	1	2	3	4	5	6	7	8	9	10
45. I just can't let it go to waste.	1	2	3	4	5	6	7	8	9	10
46. The poor starving children in . . .	1	2	3	4	5	6	7	8	9	10
47. No one will see me now, so why not.	1	2	3	4	5	6	7	8	9	10
48. I've been so good, I deserve it.	1	2	3	4	5	6	7	8	9	10
49. I might never again get a chance to eat this.	1	2	3	4	5	6	7	8	9	10
50. Well, there goes my diet; I may as well give up.	1	2	3	4	5	6	7	8	9	10
51. I always blow it when _____. (something happens)	1	2	3	4	5	6	7	8	9	10
52. After all, the holidays only come once a year.	1	2	3	4	5	6	7	8	9	10
53. I'm craving it, so my body must need it.	1	2	3	4	5	6	7	8	9	10
54. I've got to eat so I don't get a headache.	1	2	3	4	5	6	7	8	9	10
55. I was meant to be fat.	1	2	3	4	5	6	7	8	9	10
56. I'm so tired and I don't feel like cooking.	1	2	3	4	5	6	7	8	9	10

Saboteur Versus Coach Self-Talk

The Saboteur Speaking

The Coach Speaking

Procrastination

Staying Stuck

I'll start tomorrow.

Getting Unstuck

Today is the only time I've got. There are no guarantees about tomorrow. If I don't start now, I may discover my time is gone and it will be too late.

There's no use in trying.

If I don't try I'll stay stuck forever. No one can do it for me. I'm the only one who can take charge here. All I have to do is begin.

Setting Goals

Perfectionist Goals

Never again will I touch a chocolate chip cookie.

Flexible Goals

I need to learn how to eat chocolate chip cookies in moderation. Until I do I'll avoid them, but eventually I must learn to be in charge of them, instead of their being in charge of me.

From now on I'm not going to overeat.

I'm a human being and I may occasionally overeat; my job now is to make healthy food choices to avoid overeating whenever possible.

Abstract Goals

I'm going to lose 30 pounds.

Concrete Goals

To lose weight I need to focus on what I must do—exercise more, cut down on fat, reduce my drinking, etc.

Unreasonable Goals

I'm going to exercise every day.

Reasonable Goals

Next week I'll shoot to exercise at least three days, and if I do more that will be terrific.

Predicting Results

Expecting Failure

I've got so much weight to lose, there's no point in even trying.

Expecting Success

This isn't just about losing weight, it's about changing my life around and being healthier. I need to take it one step at a time, and ultimately I'll win.

I've tried before and not succeeded so why should things be different now?

Perhaps what I tried before was the wrong thing. Sometimes it takes several tries before success comes.

Saboteur Versus Coach Self-Talk

The Saboteur Speaking

The Coach Speaking

Assessing Progress

Despairing

I'm not losing weight; there must be something wrong.

Losing just a little weight each week is discouraging. (OR: I'm not losing weight fast enough.)

I'm gaining weight; I may as well quit.

No one else really cares; what's the use?

Other people are making this more difficult for me; maybe I should give up.

Encouraging

I need to reevaluate my strategy—am I cheating and getting more calories than I should, am I getting enough exercise, do I need to reduce my caloric intake even more, how can I increase my exercise?

The best way to lose weight is slow and steady. As long as I'm sure my calorie intake and exercise level are okay, I'm doing fine.

No, I need to reevaluate my strategy and make the right changes. If I keep making healthy choices, the weight will come off.

I'm doing this for me because I want to look and feel better. It would be nice if others noticed my efforts, but I don't need that to succeed.

I need to learn how to get others to support my efforts, and to deal more effectively with sabotage. I don't have to be at the mercy of others.

Coping Day-To-Day

Deprivation

Poor me, I have to give up almost everything I like.

It's not fair that others can eat what they want and I can't.

Focus on Goals

I'm retraining my tastes so that making healthy choices will be easy for me. That way, I'll have the best body I can and better health too.

I have to work with my metabolism and my needs no matter what others do. It's not fair to my body to eat inappropriately and unhealthily.

Blaming

If it weren't for my job (or my kids, or my spouse, or my mother, etc.) I could lose weight.

Sharing Responsibility

My job isn't any more demanding (or my kids, etc., aren't any more difficult) than some other people's. I just need to be more creative in finding a way to deal with this.

(continued)

Saboteur Versus Coach Self-Talk

The Saboteur Speaking

The Coach Speaking

Blaming (continued)

He (or she) keeps bringing me candy (or other tempting food), so I can't lose weight.

Sharing Responsibility (continued)

He (or she) must be doing this for a reason. Maybe I haven't been clear about what I want from him, or maybe he's feeling threatened in some way by my efforts to lose weight. I need to discuss this with him further and if necessary take stronger action to insist on my needs.

She (or he) insists that I eat.

I need to be more assertive and stand up for my well-being.

She (or he) would be offended if I didn't eat.

I'm just buying into old beliefs about being polite. Maybe I'm also assuming that she would be offended when she would not be. I need to talk with her about this so that we can both be happy.

Martyrdom

Others get bored by people who are pre-occupied with watching their weight; I am not any fun when I'm dieting.

Sharing Responsibility

Just because I'm watching my weight doesn't mean I have to be a drag. I just need to plan ahead how to participate and have fun without overeating.

It's not right to make others suffer because I want to lose weight.

Others will like me better when I like myself better.

I can't ask my children and my family to change their way of eating for me.

If I talk it over with them, they may be very supportive. After all, it's their health too.

Catastrophizing

If I don't lose weight, my family and friends will hate me.

Balanced Point of View

My family and friends may be disappointed, but they'll still love me. Besides, I'm not doing this for them; I'm doing it for me, and I've got to work it through on my own.

If I don't lose weight before going on vacation, my vacation will be ruined.

Having a good time on my vacation doesn't depend on my weight. I need to make managing weight a natural part of my life-style and stop focusing on my weight as the determinant of my happiness.

What if I slip and regain my weight; I couldn't stand it.

I may have temporary setbacks, but I need to learn to deal with these. I need to see them as something I can learn from and not evidence that I can't cope. Part of permanent success is being able to pick myself up and get going again after setbacks.

Saboteur Versus Coach Self-Talk

The Saboteur Speaking

The Coach Speaking

What if I've got too many fat cells or I'm just "naturally" fat?

That stuff about fat cells and "natural" weight may or may not be true. If it is, it doesn't mean I can't be successful. It just means that I may have to try harder.

What if this program doesn't work?

Success doesn't depend on this program. It depends on me. If I pay attention to eating correctly and getting enough exercise, with time I will succeed.

What if I don't have enough willpower?

Willpower isn't some mysterious force over which I have no control. Willpower comes from knowing what to do, thinking constructively, and taking action in small steps.

If I don't lose weight, he (she) won't love me anymore.

If being loved is dependent on my weight or my appearance, perhaps the other person has a value system I can't live with. Perhaps this is a relationship that doesn't merit my commitment to it.

Poor Self-Worth

Healthy Self-Worth

Anyone as fat as I am doesn't deserve to feel good about herself.

When I don't feel good about myself, I get depressed and look for something to eat. I need to accept myself as I am now and make a commitment to my health and well-being.

No one could like anyone as fat as I am.

Lots of overweight people are liked and respected by others. Beauty is an inner quality that comes from caring about yourself and about others, not from your physical appearance. Lots of thin, physically attractive people don't really know what beauty is, and aren't well liked.

People will love me more and my life will be better when I lose this weight.

My happiness does not depend on what I weigh. If I want more love, I have to give more love. If I am dissatisfied with certain aspects of my life, I have to face up to these problems and deal with them directly. Losing weight does not solve life's problems.

If I hate myself enough, maybe I'll change.

Belittling myself and hating myself won't motivate me to do anything except eat more. I need to be more self-accepting and focus on making healthy choices for me instead of unhealthy choices that don't serve me.

(continued)

Saboteur Versus Coach Self-Talk

The Saboteur Speaking

The Coach Speaking

Poor Self-Worth (continued)

I've never been able to please my mother (father, spouse, etc.), so why bother?

Healthy Self-Worth (continued)

It would have been nice to have my accomplishments recognized and to be appreciated by others, but it wasn't that way. Now I know that the most important evaluation of me is my self-evaluation. I'm not going to let the past hold power over me. I'm in charge now.

Focus on Temptations

Gee, wouldn't that taste good.

Refocusing and Relabeling

No, I don't want to eat that. It looks better than it tastes, I'm sure. I've had it before and it wasn't that great.

I can't handle that particular food; maybe I'm addicted to it.

No food is in charge of me, and there is no such thing as being addicted to a particular food. I have to stop thinking about and imagining the taste because that's what gets me going. I need to think about its bad qualities—so much fat. Ugh!

It smells (looks) so good—I just can't resist it.

I've got to distract my thoughts—quickly! Think about something else, and get away from this temptation as soon as possible.

I'm so hungry; I've got to eat.

Am I really hungry or is this some emotion such as anxiety that I am thinking is hunger?

I just can't stop thinking about eating.

When I let my mind hang onto images of food and thoughts about its taste, I get stuck thinking about food like a CD that keeps repeating when it gets stuck. I need to refocus on my work or a project that interests me. I need to get busy on something interesting so I won't think about eating.

I can't resist eating; I guess I'm just a compulsive eater.

Compulsive eating comes from compulsive thinking. I need to change my thoughts to something other than food.

It tasted so good; I'd really like to have more.

It's my tongue, not my tummy, that wants more. Taste is a strong motivator of overeating, bu I don't have to give in to it. I'll drink some water instead and get this temptation out of my sight as soon as possible.

Saboteur Versus Coach Self-Talk

The Saboteur Speaking

The Coach Speaking

Excuses and Rationalizations

Objective Assessment

The Saboteur Speaking	The Coach Speaking
With my schedule, it's impossible to eat right.	Schedules can pose a problem, but there is always a solution. I need to think creatively to find one. Remember, "argue for your limitations and sure enough, they're yours." I'm not going to let myself be trapped by this.
There's too much stress in my life for me to handle managing weight.	Stress is always present in life. There's never a good time to manage weight. There's only today. Using food to manage stress won't help. I need to find better ways to manage stress, including managing my time better and finding ways to stay relaxed in the face of it.
I deserve a little treat now and then.	Yes, I do deserve a treat now and then, but it doesn't have to be food. How about a bubble bath or a long walk in the woods. How can I treat myself without using food?
I paid for it; I'm going to eat it.	If you do eat it, you'll pay even more for it—in terms of self-esteem and additional effort to manage weight. Give it away, take it home, or just leave it.
I can't just let it go to waste. After all, "waste not, want not."	"Waste not, want not" is an old saying that that made sense once, but doesn't make sense any more. Let go of old ideas.
The poor starving children in . . .	My eating won't help any starving children anywhere. This was just a guilt trip laid on me as a child to get me to eat.
No one will see me now, so why not?	No one will see me, but I'll know. Just because no one sees me doesn't mean the calories don't count. Who am I tricking anyway? Me! I'm the one who pays the price. Why not find something else to occupy my time when I'm alone, or call someone to be with me.
I've been so good, I deserve it.	I do deserve to celebrate, but I don't have to do it with food. I can treat myself by doing something nice—like buying myself a blouse or arranging to get a massage.
I might never again get a chance to eat this.	True, but I'll also forget it quickly. If I do eat it, the pounds will be with me a lot longer than the taste.

(continued)

Saboteur Versus Coach Self-Talk

The Saboteur Speaking	The Coach Speaking
Excuses and Rationalizations (continued) Well, there goes my diet; I may as well give up.	*Objective Assessment (continued)* A temporary setback does not have to signal full blown backsliding. Just be cause I slipped doesn't mean I should give up. I need to pick myself up immediately and renew my efforts.
I always blow it on weekends.	Weekends are difficult for me, but I don't have to blow it. I can take charge by planning ahead how to handle them differently.
The holidays only come once a year.	Even "once a year" isn't a good excuse to pig out. I can plan ahead how to enjoy myself without overdoing.
I'm craving it, so my body must need it.	My body doesn't "crave" anything; my mind does. I need to change the focus of my thoughts to avoid cravings. I also need to make sure I am eating regularly and making healthy choices.
I've got to eat so I won't get a headache.	Preventative eating is an excuse based on fear, not reality. If I'm eating regularly and making healthy choices, I won't get a headache. If I do start to get a headache, it's more likely from poor stress management, and that's where I need to focus my efforts.
I was meant to be fat.	Genes are not destiny. I can overcome even a biological tendency to fatness by adopting a healthy lifestyle.
I'm so tired, and I don't feel like cooking.	I'll have a glass of juice as a pick-me-up and relax with a hot bath or a nice walk. Then I'll be in a better frame of mind to fix dinner.
I feel fat and ugly, so I must be fat and ugly; I may as well eat!	When I'm feeling down, I often conclude it's because I'm fat, when it's really because other things are getting to me. I can check myself on the scale to see if I've gained weight, or I can do something nice for myself other than eating.

(text continued from page 52)

given in the column labeled "The Coach Speaking." The statement suggested in this column may or may not work for you. If it does, adopt it. If it doesn't, develop your own counterargument that does.

Using a Double Column Technique

The *Saboteur vs. Coach Self-Talk* section (pages 56–62) that you just read is an example of a double column technique. In the left column is listed the examples of negative self-talk; in the right column are suggested counterarguments. You should make up your own double column table to help you identify your negative self-talk and construct the counterarguments you can use against such self-talk.

Draw a line down the center of a piece of paper. Label the left column, "Negative Self-Talk," and the right column, "Positive Self-Talk." Use the table given in Chapter 1 (page 12) to help you identify your own negative self-talk, and also refer to the *Saboteur vs. Coach Self-Talk* section given in this chapter. It may also be helpful to refer to the *Benefits and Costs Analysis* form you completed in Chapter 2.

In the left column, write down the things you typically say to yourself that undermine your weight management efforts. In the right column write down the counterarguments or positive things you might say instead. Give careful thought to these. You may find you need to rework a counterargument several times to get it right. It may be helpful to reread the categories of positive self-talk given in the table in Chapter 1 to help you here.

Thought Stopping

Whenever you find yourself thinking any thoughts from the left column, you can use the technique of "thought stopping." That is, think to yourself, "Stop!" and immediately dismiss the negative thought and focus your attention on the counterargument or positive thought you have developed to compete with that negative thought. You will probably have to do this again and again before the positive thought takes hold. (Some people find that wearing a rubber band on their wrist and snapping it against their skin at the same time they think "Stop!" helps to refocus their attention.)

Thought stopping involves learning to switch from negative thoughts that are upsetting or self-defeating to positive thoughts and images that are supportive and calming. This technique can be particularly helpful in overcoming racing thoughts, or the feeling of being overwhelmed by ideas and worries that seem to be uncontrollably crowding into your mind.

Before beginning this exercise, take some time to develop self-talk that will help you cope with upset, as well as a pleasurable mental image you can call up when you feel stressed. An example of coping self-talk might be, "Okay relax. Everything's fine. You can handle it. Just focus on breathing and relaxing."

A coping mental image might be a memory of a place you have been and where you felt really relaxed, calm, happy, or at peace. An example might be watching a beautiful sunset at the beach, or sitting quietly by a mountain stream and listening to the sounds of the forest. Or it might be an image of yourself doing something you enjoy, such as seeing and feeling yourself skiing down a snow-covered trail.

To make sure you can bring this image into your mind with as much vividness as possible, practice it several times beforehand. Really focus on "seeing" the details of the scene, "sensing" the experience, and feeling relaxed.

Thought Stopping Exercise

Once you have your coping self-talk and you are able to mentally transport yourself to a relaxing place, you can practice the following exercise for using thought stopping:

1. First, find a quiet, private place, get comfortable, close your eyes, and intentionally let thoughts enter your mind that have upset you in the past or that you find yourself brooding about at times. Let these thoughts and images flood your mind until you are beginning to feel uneasy, perhaps even a little anxious.

2. When you get to a level of uneasiness or discomfort that is mild but not too intense, shout out loud the word, "STOP!" You might also clap your hands or hit the table with your fist at the same time—the intention being to startle yourself and actually short-circuit your thinking and terminate the depressing thought. Or you might snap a rubber band on your wrist, or pinch yourself.

3. Immediately switch your thinking to the coping self-talk you have constructed ahead of time. At the same time, take some deep breaths, and let yourself relax. Now bring to mind as vividly as possible the relaxing and calming mental image you practiced earlier. Let your body relax and let go of the tension you felt during the negative thinking.

4. If you were able to completely relax, go on to the next step. If you found yourself still bothered by the negative thoughts from step one, you probably let yourself become too upset during step one. Repeat step one, but this time interrupt the negative thoughts sooner. Do this until you can relax and let go completely at step three.

5.   Repeat this thought stopping exercise, but this time allow yourself to *think* "STOP!" to yourself, instead of shouting it out loud. Do not snap the rubber band or pinch yourself this time. Follow this with deep breaths, coping self-talk, and a pleasant mental image. Allow your body to relax as in step three.

Repeat this step as often as necessary until you are able to both mentally and physically relax and let go after negative thinking.

6.   Practice the technique several times, thinking "STOP!" to yourself and keeping the level of arousal low to moderate, before trying to use it in an actual problem situation. After you have mastered thought stopping with these steps, you should be able to use the technique at any time you are confronted with upsetting thoughts.

Remember, the technique works best if used in the beginning, when the unwanted thoughts are just starting and before the emotional arousal gets too high.

Developing More Positive Self-Talk

In addition to replacing negative self-talk with positive self-talk, and learning how to thought stop when necessary, you need to learn how to use self-talk to keep yourself on track and focused on success. Part of your natural thinking process involves giving yourself instructions and reminders about what you need to do, and taking note of your progress.

In fact, you do this all the time, whether you realize it or not. The example given at the beginning of this chapter shows how instructional self-talk may be involved in finding lost keys.

But when emotions get out of hand, self-instructional thoughts may give way to panic thinking or angry self-blaming. Emotional thinking can disrupt good decision making and cloud the objective assessment of the situation. Learning to keep emotions under control and to focus on what needs to be done are important for smart thinking.

Self-instructional statements are particularly useful for coping with situations that are potentially stressful and that can be anticipated. An example of such a situation would be having to go through your yearly job performance review. For several days or weeks before the review, you are likely to be worried and nervous about it—so much so that you may start nibbling or snacking inappropriately to try and push away the anxiety. By the time the actual interview takes place, you may be so anxious that you don't do as well in the interview as you might have. Then, whether the review turns out good or bad, afterwards you may attempt to soothe your still-frazzled nerves with something "yummy" to eat.

Stress Inoculation

Self-instructional self-talk is the basis for a powerful technique for managing stress. When you know that a potentially stressful situation is in the offing, you need to use the technique of stress inoculation.[3] This involves preparing and using instructional self-statements, as well as mentally rehearsing how you will act and feel during an impending stressful situation.

To prepare for successful stress-inoculation, you need to break a situation into three stages: the *Before Stage*, when you are preparing for the situation; the *During Stage*, when you must actually cope with it; and the *After Stage*, when you must deal with any residual arousal and stress.

You need to plan what you will mentally say to yourself during each of these stages. Be sure to plan self-talk that focuses on controlling your physical arousal, that directs you in what to do, and that reminds you of how well you are doing.

To help you understand this better, consider how one woman did this very successfully. Nancy had had an argument with her daughter, and now she was anticipating making a telephone call to the daughter to try and make up. She used the stress inoculation technique to cope with the stress before, during, and after the telephone conversation.

She planned to telephone her daughter and invite her to come visit for the holidays. She did not know whether the daughter would accept, so she had to be prepared for a rejection. Consider the mental image and self-talk that Nancy rehearsed for each stage.

Before Stage

With hand on the telephone, ready to make the call, Nancy thinks to herself:

- It will be all right.

- No matter whether she accepts, she'll know I care.

- If she doesn't accept, it doesn't mean she doesn't love me.

- Now, take some deep breaths.

- Relax.

- Keep your voice calm and friendly. Good, you'll be okay.

During Stage

Nancy is actually speaking with her daughter and at the same time thinking to herself:

- You're doing fine.

- Keep calm, it will be okay.

- Keep your voice even; don't show irritation. Stay relaxed.

- She sounds fine.

- Whatever choice she makes is okay. Smile with your voice.

- Tell her you love her.

- Good.

After Stage

Nancy has hung up the phone and is thinking to herself:

- You did fine.

- She got the message that you love her, and that's what you wanted most.

- Take some deep breaths. Relax. Let's go for a walk and get a breath of fresh air.

Having imagined the scene and rehearsed her self-talk, Nancy was better able to stay calm during the actual phone call and keep herself focused on what she wanted to accomplish. In fact, Nancy mentally rehearsed various scenarios of how the situation might turn out. She was prepared for either acceptance or refusal, and the self-instructional statements she planned to use helped her do the best she could and calmly accept the outcome.

To use self-instructional statements to manage the stress associated with some potentially distressing situation, use the following planning sheet to create the self-talk you will use. Create some statements that will help you stay focused on the task at hand or on the actions you need to take to stay on track, and create others that will help you manage your emotional arousal at each stage. Then imagine yourself going through the entire situation from start to finish, including imagining what you will say to yourself at each of the stages. Stay calm and relaxed during this mental rehearsal, and repeat it several times to maximize your ability to cope with it most effectively.

Talking Yourself Into Success

With positive self-talk, you can literally talk yourself into success. Here are some more tips for getting control of your thinking and your self-talk.

Getting Over Procrastination

If you are a procrastinator, you tend to be very rational. You have lots of neat, little explanations and excuses to justify why you can't, shouldn't, or couldn't take action now. As a procrastinator, you are very good at denying the facts,

Stress Inoculation Planning Form

Description of a potentially stressful situation: _____

_____

_____

Action Statements	**Emotion-Managing Statements**
Before Stage	
During Stage	
After Stage	

or distorting information so that you don't have to take action. Often you are invested in being right about your inaction because:

> . . . you don't or won't see a solution to your situation, or the solutions that are available are not ones you want to try,

> . . . you have created excuses or rationalizations that keep you stuck,

> . . . you feel overwhelmed or trapped, or

> . . . you are still focusing on the costs to you of trying to lose weight, and/or the benefits you get from not bothering.

To get unstuck and get moving, you need to realize that you keep yourself stuck by what you say to yourself. When you focus on "I can't," it's guaranteed you won't. When you focus on "I will," you open the possibility of finding an acceptable solution that wasn't apparent when you were still insisting that you couldn't.

Start thinking creatively. Usually nothing worth having is acquired without some effort. You may have barriers to overcome, but you are the only one who can overcome them. Remind yourself that if you wait too long to take action, some day it may be too late. The longer you wait, the harder it will be to get started and succeed.

Perhaps you have some good reasons for not getting started. It may seem that your life is particularly stressful, and that it is all you can do just to cope with life day to day. That may be true, but it is also true that life is a series of crises interspersed with relatively calm spaces. Like a roller coaster—there are peaks and there are depths. Depending on how you let yourself feel about it, the ride can be frightening or exhilarating.

There is never a really "good" time to start a weight management effort. Even once you do start, some life crisis is likely to materialize during the process. You must learn to cope with the crisis at the same time. Indeed, the changes in your thinking, your behavior, and your lifestyle that you will be making are likely to make it easier for you to handle the crisis when it does come.

If you are feeling overwhelmed, you need to take a problem-solving approach, and break the solution into small, manageable steps, rather than trying to tackle the whole thing at once. Focus on accomplishing each small step, and don't get discouraged by the enormity of the project.

If you need to lose 100 pounds, think in terms of losing ten pounds at a time. Focus on making and maintaining small behavior changes each day. Count up your little daily wins, rather than waiting till you reach goal weight to declare yourself a winner. Remind yourself daily that you are making progress, and that you are pleased with yourself. Remember that a journey of a thousand miles begins with the first step. Then take it one day at a time, one step at a time.

If you are still focusing on what you have to lose by making the weight loss effort, and are not too sure that what you have to gain is worth it, review the *Benefits and Costs Analysis* that you completed earlier. If you are still stuck in procrastination, you may need to redo this analysis, or at least to refocus your attention to the unshaded boxes. Refer to your *Benefits and Costs Analysis,* and create self-talk that will keep you focused on the benefits you have to gain by losing weight, and the costs you are paying or will pay by not reducing.

Setting Appropriate Goals

In reviewing your *Benefits and Costs Analysis* from Chapter 1, you may discover that the benefits you expect to get by losing weight are unrealistic. Losing weight may not help you find the love of your life, and you may still be stuck in the same old job. Be sure the goal you are striving to reach by losing weight is realistic. Stop telling yourself that "life will be better when I lose weight." Concentrate on making life good now *and* making the healthy choices that will lead to the best body you can have.

It is also possible that the benefits you initially wanted to get from losing weight are not really as important as you thought in the beginning. Perhaps they are benefits that someone else thinks are important. You need to find reasons for losing weight that are meaningful to you. These reasons must also be important enough to you to offset the effort you must make to achieve long-term success.

Perhaps you got involved in weight management because someone else wants you to lose weight, but losing weight is less important to you. You need to want to lose weight for yourself. When someone else pressures you to do so, and you are doing it for them more than for yourself, your chances for success will be very small.

Once you are sure your long-term goals are appropriate, focus on setting appropriate, short-term goals. Avoid setting abstract goals, such as, "I want to lose 30 pounds." Set specific, concrete, behavioral goals such as, "I will increase my exercise to 30 minutes a day, five days a week, and I'll maintain a caloric intake of 1200 to 1400 a day."

Don't set yourself up for failure by insisting on perfection. Beware of resolutions that include the words "never" or "always." Establishing a goal containing these words is a sure-fire ticket to failure. Leave room to make mistakes or deviate somewhat, because human beings are not perfect. Set up a reasonable objective that you have a good chance of reaching, such as, "I'll exercise at least three days a week," and then be pleased if you do more.

Revising Expectations

When you fail at something once, you are likely to develop an expectation that you will fail again. Often this is because you decide that it was your fault, that something you did or didn't do made it turn out that way. A more objective analysis might show that other factors played an equally important role. Perhaps the approach you tried was inadequate. Perhaps an unexpected stressful situation came up that disrupted your efforts.

You need to challenge the notion that it was all your fault, and the logical extension of that notion—that you won't be successful in the future either. Tell yourself that this time is different. You can succeed by focusing on making long-term changes and doing it one step at a time.

Focusing on Progress

Be sure you are using appropriate measures to judge progress. Focusing only on what the scale says is inappropriate. The scale can mislead you into thinking you are making great progress when in fact you are losing fluid, or that you are not making much progress when in fact you are. You need additional ways to measure progress.

Observing yourself make progress in changing behavior, increasing exercise, and choosing food differently are all important ways to judge success. Noticing differences in the way your clothes fit is also helpful. You will get yourself into trouble with motivation if you make reaching goal weight the only evidence of your success. You must have lots of intermediate measures of success, and then you must give yourself credit for accomplishing them.

At the end of each day, take a few moments to review your successes for the day. What did you accomplish? What did you do well at? Where can you improve tomorrow? Pat yourself on the back, and encourage yourself to keep up the good work (or to pick yourself up and start again).

Ensuring Sufficient Rewards

Every person needs to have some rewards and some pleasure in life. You need to nurture yourself every day. If the only way you nurture yourself is to eat, you will have great difficulty managing your weight. Review the way you live your life and notice how you reward yourself. If food and eating is about your only pleasure, you need to think creatively about other ways to nurture yourself.

Taking some time each day to contribute to your physical pleasure is a good start—plan a nice walk each day, or a bubble bath, or a massage, or a nap.

When the baby goes to sleep, put on a dance exercise tape and indulge your body in some fun and relaxing exercise. (Don't give into the temptation to numb your mind with a soap opera—that's not pleasure for your body.) Try putting a number of ideas for physical pleasure on different slips of paper in a "reward box." Each day, draw out a slip to see what you get to do for yourself that day. Remember to tell yourself that you deserve a little pleasure for your body each day.

When you have lots of ways to reward and nurture yourself, you are less likely to feel deprived. Feelings of deprivation arise partly from lack of sufficient rewards and partly from the way you think. Declaring some food off limits or "illegal" is likely to contribute to feelings of deprivation, leading you to focus on that food and to talk to yourself about how it's "not fair," or how you deserve a treat now and then.

Instead of declaring a food bad or forbidden, tell yourself that it is not a particularly healthy choice, and that while you may eat it now and then, you prefer to make healthy choices for your body. (After all, if it were your pet, wouldn't you make sure it got the healthy choice. Doesn't your body deserve at least as good consideration and treatment as your pet?)

When you know you may make any food choice you like, and you focus on making the choice that is the healthy one, you avoid the restrictive "dieter's mentality." To do so, nurture yourself with nonfood rewards, and focus on making the healthy choices your body deserves.

Sharing Responsibility

Blaming others or forces outside yourself for the actions you take is a distortion, one that fails to take into account how your own beliefs and behavior contributed. You may blame others for your eating because of your beliefs about politeness or social niceties. You may make excuses for yourself by blaming others, when in fact you could find a solution if you chose to be creative. Perhaps you don't communicate your needs to others assertively, or in such a way that they understand and act appropriately.

Rather than seeing yourself as a victim, which defines you as having no power to change things and keeps you stuck, consider how you share in the responsibility for your actions. Focus on what you can do to change things, rather than on why it wasn't your fault.

The opposite side of blaming others involves blaming yourself completely, or allowing yourself to be a martyr for someone else. As a martyr you hold beliefs about what is "right" and appropriate behavior, believing, for example, that it is not "right" to seek assistance or support from others, that it is "right" to do it all yourself, that it isn't "right" to burden others with your problems, and so forth. You may think you bear the major responsibility for other people's happiness and that your own needs should only be addressed after the needs of others are met.

All people live in a network of family, friends, and acquaintances, and all share in the responsibility of getting needs met. To do this, people need to communicate with one another about needs and be willing to ask for support. A balance needs to be struck between expecting others to take care of you, and bearing the entire burden yourself.

In your self-talk, remind yourself that both you and your loved ones share in the responsibility for getting needs met fairly. Are you doing all you can for yourself, including asking for the support of others? Acknowledging the necessity of shared responsibility, and taking steps to ensure it is an important step in creating successful long-term weight management.

Developing a Balanced Point of View

If your self-talk is filled with "what ifs" and alarmist thoughts, you may be in the bad habit of catastrophizing. One woman called this the "Jewish mother" way of thinking. You need to develop the habit of taking a more balanced point of view.

Instead of focusing on the possibility of disaster, get some distance between yourself and the problem. Imagine that you can climb into a helicopter and go up several hundred feet until you can look down upon the problem. Such a vantage point often makes things look different, and finding an appropriate solution is more likely when you can put some distance between yourself and the problem.

Avoid letting emotions run away with you. Catastrophizing leads to "panic" thinking—the same thoughts race repeatedly through your head and your ability to think of solutions is reduced. When you find yourself in this situation, use the thought stopping technique you learned on page 64. Ask yourself, "What would I tell a friend who was in this situation and needed sound advice?" Then take your own advice.

Developing a Healthy Self-Worth

People naturally look to others for acceptance. When others are rejecting or negative, you may take this as entirely a reflection on you, leading you to lowered self-esteem, and never realize that the rejection or negative evaluation is more likely to be a statement about the other person than about you. Often people are critical of you because they see something of themselves in you, or in some way you represent a threat to them. Or they may have a rigid set of beliefs about the way things ought and ought not to be.

Developing and maintaining a healthy sense of self-worth involves reminding yourself of this, and encouraging self-acceptance of yourself. Self-acceptance means acknowledging truthfully your imperfections and your good qualities, and accepting the things about you that you cannot change.

Some people are afraid that self-acceptance will lead to inaction—to not trying to change bad habits. On the contrary, belittling and criticizing yourself will not motivate change—it will motivate an attempt to feel better, and that might mean getting something to eat so you can feel good.

Instead, remind yourself that this is the only body you are going to get, and you want to take the very best care of it and nurture it. Remember, you are not your body, but you are not separate from it either. You need your body, so take care of it as you would a prized possession.

Refocusing and Relabeling

When you give in to temptation, it is because your focus has shifted to the rewards to be gotten from what is tempting you. Any notions about why you shouldn't give in to the temptation are usually dismissed or discounted with your self-talk.

What you need is to refocus on the rewards for resisting temptation, and the costs of giving in to it. It also helps to relabel the temptation—instead of thinking about how "good" it is, think about the negative aspects. Likewise, you can relabel a cost. Instead of experiencing hunger as "bad," think of hunger pangs as meaning that you are losing weight, and rejoice in them.

By relabeling, you can literally retrain your taste buds by constantly telling yourself you don't like one particular food and do like another. Right now, you are probably reinforcing your present taste preferences by telling yourself things such as, "Gee, that taste's so good," "I just love chocolate," "I can't resist ice cream," "I hate fruit," and so forth. You can reverse this, just by talking to yourself in the opposite way, and doing so for a long enough period of time.

Refuting Justifications to Indulge or Backslide

Excuses and rationalizations are "perfectly logical" reasons that you create for yourself by distorting or denying the facts. You use them to justify an indulgence, or to allow yourself to backslide into old habits.

You distort information that comes to you, in a variety of ways. You may only pay attention to certain features and ignore others. Thus, you recall that some weekends have proven especially difficult for managing weight, and forget to remember that there have been weekends when you have done well. This selective recall leads you to throw up your hands and not even try to succeed on weekends.

Or you may focus on the small setback you have just had, and conclude that there is no use, instead of putting this one into perspective and remembering that you have made a lot of progress too. You need to develop a more balanced point of view, and remind yourself of this in your self-talk.

Often, excuses and rationalizations are built upon beliefs and notions that are out of date or not applicable. You may have grown up in an era or in a family that advocated certain ideas, like "women shouldn't exercise," or "good girls take care of others." When you don't challenge these beliefs, they will generate self-talk that undermines your chances of success.

Refuting justifications to indulge or backslide involves noticing your tendencies to distort or deny the facts, paying attention to all of the relevant information, challenging beliefs and ideas that no longer apply, and creating strong counter-arguments with which to confront excuses and rationalizations.

Summary

Self-talk is conscious thinking. What you say to yourself—your self-talk—influences how you feel and what you do. Some kinds of self-talk help you cope better and achieve your goals. This is called "positive" self-talk. On the other hand, negative self-talk is self-defeating, because it undermines your motivation and hinders coping behavior. When your negative self-talk outweighs the amount of positive self-talk, your chances of success are reduced.

The key to long-term success in managing weight is to increase positive self-talk and reduce negative self-talk.

References

1.   Schwartz, R.M. (1986). The internal dialogue: On the asymmetry between positive and negative coping thoughts. *Cognitive Therapy and Research, 10,* 591–605.

2.   Schwartz, R.M., & Garamoni, G.L. (1986). A structural model of positive and negative states of mind: Asymmetry in the internal dialogue. *Advances in Cognitive-Behavioral Research and Therapy, 5,* 2–55.

3.   Meichenbaum, D., & Cameron, R. (1983). Stress inoculation training: Toward a general paradigm for training coping skills. In D. Meichenbaum & M.E. Jaremko (Eds.), *Stress Reduction and Prevention.* New York: Plenum Press (pp. 115–154).

Chapter 5

Coping With
Social Influences

*TWO WOMEN were standing before a pastry display case. The over-*weight woman said to the thinner woman:

"I'll have one if you will."

"I don't think so," replied the other.

"Oh, come on, just split one with me."

"No," replied the thinner woman, "It's been a real struggle to get to goal weight, and I want to stay there." The overweight woman tried harder:

"Come on. You're so thin, you can afford a little treat. Besides, having half of mine isn't so bad." The thinner woman looked as though she would waver and obviously was perplexed.

"No, I won't," she finally said with conviction. "I just don't eat that way anymore. If I'm going to spend my calories, I want it to be for something I really want."

At that point, a third person who was overhearing this conversation said:

"Good for you." With a broad smile and a flush of embarrassment, the thinner woman said:

"Thanks, I needed that."

Social Influences

Everyone is subject to social influences—the subtle and sometimes not so subtle pressures that others exert to get you to behave in certain ways. Weight management does not take place independently of others around you. Family, friends, co-workers, acquaintances, and people just in general influence how you think, feel, and act.

People whose values you share and opinions you respect exert the most influence on your beliefs and actions, but even strangers can have an impact on your behavior. To get to goal weight and to stay there involves being able to cope with these social influences, and to make them work for you whenever possible.

Perhaps you resist the idea of getting help from others. You may believe you "should be able" to do it all yourself. Or like the woman who used a succession of aliases to join Weight Watchers repeatedly, you may feel that you "should have licked" this problem a long time ago, and you don't want others to know you are trying yet again. A crucial aspect of permanent success is involving others effectively in your efforts, and developing the skills to manage the inevitable social influences that affect your eating and your exercise behavior.

Often others who don't have a weight problem don't understand the difficulty of managing weight, and the personal trauma that can be involved when weight is regained after so much effort has been made to lose it. Some people think that having difficulty with weight is the result of some kind of "personality problem." Others can be very judgmental, and you may worry that regaining some of the weight you lost will lead them to make comments such as, "How could you let yourself go like that?"

Some people offer well-meaning advice or simplistic solutions, such as, "just push yourself away from the table." Equally disheartening is the person who says nothing, but who lets you know nonverbally they are watching—and judging—what you do.

Even people who know the difficulties involved in managing weight often do not recognize how their actions can undermine your efforts—or if they do, they may not want to admit it. The overweight woman who wanted her friend to share a pastry probably did not mean to sabotage her friend's success; she just wanted justification for her own actions. People who urge you to overeat may genuinely want you to enjoy some pleasure, and believe that you will be grateful for their efforts.

Getting Support, Not Sabotage

Sometimes people try to help, but their efforts backfire. The spouse or friend who constantly watches what you eat and makes comments on your efforts may intend to be helpful, but instead may cause you to feel anxious or angry, or to rebel and eat inappropriately just to get back at them.

When someone watches you critically, it can be as harmful as someone not giving you credit for your efforts. The trick is to get others to support your efforts without inadvertently sabotaging you.

Sometimes those around you see their lives being altered by your weight management efforts, and they resist the changes that are involved. Changing your way of eating usually causes others to have to eat differently. They may react negatively when challenged to make health changes themselves.

One couple, Colleen and Carl, discovered this when Colleen undertook her weight management effort. She changed her way of cooking and refused to prepare fancy desserts. Carl, who enjoyed eating high-fat food, felt punished and judged by Colleen. He knew he should lose some weight too, and it seemed to him that Colleen was giving him a not-so-subtle message that he should change his habits. He reacted with anger and resistance to her weight management efforts.

Feeling as if change is being "forced" on one can create anger or anxiety, and this can lead to sabotage. Sabotage can take many forms. It may involve the other person's bringing you gifts of food, offering you high-calorie food, or simply leaving food around for you to find. It may involve the other person's wanting impulsively to stop at a fast food restaurant where you can only get high-fat, high-calorie foods.

To cope with this kind of sabotage you need to develop and use skills in communicating assertively. Speak up. Ask for the other person's cooperation. Be willing to say "no" and stick to it. Work on finding a compromise that will meet some of everyone's needs.

Sabotage may sound like someone saying to you, "You've already lost enough weight, now you're too thin," or "I liked you better when you had a little meat on your bones." When someone you care about makes such statements, it is often because that person is afraid that you are too attractive to others, and he or she might lose you to someone else. Sometimes, that person sees your having lost weight as a threat to their influence over you.

Taking care to assure others, and to talk openly and honestly about the problem is the way to deal with these types of situations. If left unattended, the other person's feelings and behavior can play havoc with your weight management success.

Sometimes sabotage results from culturally-based beliefs about what is good or acceptable. Sometimes because of a particular ethnic or racial background, families in which most of the members are overweight tend to see their normal weight members as too thin, and they put pressure on them to "get some meat on those bones." Fatness tends to be more acceptable in some groups, and is even seen as a sign of good health or status. In such situations, resisting or challenging cultural ideas about what is "good" or "right" concerning food, eating, and weight can be difficult; but it is essential for long-term success.

Involving others in your weight management efforts in a way that is non-threatening to them is important if you are going to stay at your best weight.

Many times, however, you sabotage yourself. Even though it seems that social influences are to blame, beliefs you hold and assumptions you make can lead you to feel obligated to eat at times you would otherwise consider inappropriate.

When Carl brought Colleen candy and sweets, she felt she shouldn't hurt her husband's feelings by refusing them. If you feel it "isn't right" to refuse to eat something that someone has brought or prepared especially for you, even though it isn't in your best interests, you are setting yourself up for problems. When you fail to communicate effectively about what you want and need from others to support your weight management efforts, you set yourself up for problems.

Yet another way to sabotage yourself, while thinking you are helping yourself, is to get someone to play "watchdog" for you. You may ask someone to call your attention to inappropriate eating, to remind you to stay on track. Unfortunately, this makes the other person responsible for your behavior, and may even set him or her up for taking blame.

Elsie got into trouble this way when she asked her husband to help her cope with eating at a party they were going to. He obliged by giving her stern looks when she took another helping, and even took some food away from her. She got so upset by his constant surveillance that she had an eating binge when they got home from the party.

Betty played the watchdog game another way. She asked a friend to help her manage her eating, and then regularly tested to see if the friend was indeed watching. Betty also noted whether her friend was sufficiently tactful in admonishing her when she slipped, and felt hurt when she perceived less tact than she thought appropriate. In fact, Betty was testing to see whether or not the friend really cared for her. Because of her hidden agenda, it was assured that Betty would eat inappropriately.

When you have rigid ideas about what your proper role is and how you "should" behave, you expose yourself to social influences that seem out of your control. For example, holding beliefs about how a "successful" business person must entertain clients with food and drink, or how a "good" hostess is expected to serve fancy (i.e., high-calorie) food, is a form of self-sabotage. When you set up these sorts of situations, and then make up excuses that allow you to eat too, you are not merely subject to social influences, you are involved in self-sabotage as well.

To effectively cope with social influences, you must examine the beliefs and assumptions you hold about what is right and proper behavior and, if necessary, change the way you think. You need to distinguish between the times when you are in fact the problem, and the times when others are the problem. You need to develop specific skills for coping with certain social influences, and bring to bear techniques that have been shown to work.

Social influence by definition comes from outside yourself, but it affects you only to the extent that your thinking and your ability to respond and cope effectively allow it to influence you.

How to Cope With Social Influences

Beliefs and Social Influences

Coping with social influences begins with becoming more aware of and challenging the beliefs and assumptions that keep you stuck. Complete the self-test on page 81 to determine what your "pressure quotient" is—the extent to which you hold onto beliefs that make you more susceptible to social influences that undermine your weight management efforts.

Challenging Your Beliefs and Assumptions

If you don't believe you have the right to say no to someone, or if you feel it isn't polite to refuse food when it is offered, if you assume you will hurt the other person's feelings by refusing, or if you are afraid to speak up for your own needs, you will have an extremely difficult time coping with social influences.

You *do* have the right to refuse, even if the other person is really in need, or if the other person means well, just as the other person also has the right to refuse you. If he takes offense at your refusal, this is because of his beliefs about how you should act, and not because you really did something wrong.

But you can learn how to say no in such a way that the other person is less likely to be offended, and so that he or she is more likely to clearly understand that you really mean no when you say it. What is more, if you anticipate the situation and discuss your needs beforehand, the problem is likely to be avoided entirely.

If you assume that your spouse or family will not want to be included in your weight management efforts, you may inadvertently create resentment in those you care about; they may feel left out, or may interpret your actions as "not wanting" their help. By not checking this out with them, you close off the possibility of their support, and this can be crucial. Let them know what you are trying to do, and exactly what you would like them to do to support you (such as, "notice when I'm doing well but don't notice when I'm not," or "don't cook fattening dishes for me when I visit").

Holding onto restricting ideas about what is required of you can make weight management difficult. Some business people claim that entertaining clients presents a problem, because clients expect to be "wined and dined," and the business person must order drinks and a big entree in order to allow clients to feel comfortable about what they order. This ignores the fact that a business person is more successful when he or she can relate to clients on a genuine and honest level. Putting on a "show" usually creates a negative impression.

It would be better to state your intention to order mineral water, and invite the client to feel free to order what he likes. (Sometimes this takes pressure off the client to order alcohol that he also doesn't really want.) You

Self-Test 5.1

What Is Your "Pressure Quotient"?

Rate yourself on each of the following statements according to how much you agree or disagree with each one. When you have rated yourself on all statements, add up the total points to determine your "pressure quotient." A score interpretation follows page 82.

	Strongly Disagree				Strongly Agree
1. It's not right to say "no" when someone is just trying to be nice to me.	1	2	3	4	5
2. It isn't polite to refuse food when someone has prepared it especially for me.	1	2	3	4	5
3. It's often hard for me to speak up for what I need or want.	1	2	3	4	5
4. I'd rather put my own needs second than hurt someone else's feelings.	1	2	3	4	5
5. It isn't fair to want others to help me in my weight management efforts.	1	2	3	4	5
6. I shouldn't involve others in my problems.	1	2	3	4	5
7. I need to order drinks or a "big" entree at a restaurant in order to make my clients feel comfortable.	1	2	3	4	5
8. When someone else is paying for it, I feel I may as well take advantage.	1	2	3	4	5
9. Guests that are invited to dinner expect to be treated to fancy (which generally means "high-calorie") meals.	1	2	3	4	5
10. A good host or hostess fixes special meals for company, and this usually involves sauces, a high-fat entree, and perhaps a sugary dessert.	1	2	3	4	5
11. When invited to dinner, I should show my appreciation by eating well.	1	2	3	4	5
12. Calling ahead to inquire about the menu, or making special requests of a hostess whom I know, is making a nuisance of myself and I shouldn't do it.	1	2	3	4	5
13. Other people depend on me, and their needs must come first.	1	2	3	4	5
14. When someone tries to pressure me, I resist, even if what they want me to do is a good idea.	1	2	3	4	5
15. When someone I care about doesn't want me to change, I feel I shouldn't try to change.	1	2	3	4	5
16. I like the sympathy and attention I get from having a weight problem.	1	2	3	4	5
17. When I see others eating, I just can't resist getting something to eat too.	1	2	3	4	5
18. I can't resist food at parties and celebrations that involve food.	1	2	3	4	5

Total Score   ___+___+___+___+___=___

Score Interpretation

54-90—High "Pressure Quotient"
Much of your belief system makes it harder for you to cope with social influences. You need to challenge your beliefs and make changes in the way you think.

37-53—Moderate "Pressure Quotient"
Some of your beliefs make it difficult for you to cope with social influences. Identify which beliefs keep you stuck, and change your way of thinking on these.

18-36—Low "Pressure Quotient"
Your beliefs stand you in good stead to resist social influences.

---

might comment on your new-found resolve to make "healthy choices" when it comes to ordering the entree, or you might simply make your own choice and let the client order whatever he chooses without further comment.

Alternatively, you might invite the client to order first, so that he won't be influenced by what you do. In fact, "needing to make the client feel comfortable" is often a rationalization that covers up another notion that is really influencing your behavior—the thought that "I can write it off, so why not enjoy it."

Role Obligations

With the increased concern about health, many guests would prefer that hosts and hostesses serve "lighter" meals, but old-fashioned ideas about what makes a good host or hostess (and guests happy) still prevail—and sabotage weight management. Serving "lighter" and healthier meals may mean trying out untested recipes, or making the extra effort to cook a new way. It is usually easier to fall back on old favorites—meals that have gotten rave reviews in the past—than to risk a new menu that may not turn out. To be permanently successful with weight management means changing the way you cook (and the way you think about cooking and entertaining), not only for yourself, but for your guests as well.

As a guest, there are a variety of things you can do to ensure that the host or hostess feels free to prepare a "lighter" and healthier meal. Rather than calling ahead and asking them to avoid cooking a high-fat meal, call ahead and encourage them to avoid going to great trouble to fix the usual "heavy" guest meal, and to feel free to serve a "light" entree.

It's all in the way you phrase it—if you are positive and upbeat, rather than negative and limiting in the way you make the request, the host or hostess is likely to respond positively (and gratefully). Take the lead; offer to bring a dish, or make a specific suggestion of some dish that is "light" and healthy.

In order to speak up for your needs, you may need to challenge and change old ideas. Lynne grew up with the traditional picture that a wife and mother's obligation was to take care of the children while the husband earned a living. To ask for her husband's help caring for the children while she attended an exercise program seemed unfair to him and that she was shirking her obligations. To make time for exercise meant first challenging her assumptions about her role and about what was fair, and then taking appropriate action.

Cultural Norms and Values

When the people with whom you identify most strongly hold certain ideas or values, it is very difficult to resist this influence. Carmen cooked traditional Mexican food just as her mother had, and her family liked it that way. Making even small changes, such as replacing lard with polyunsaturated oil, was difficult because of the cultural pressure to cook in traditional ways.

In families where nearly everyone is obese, fatness is often perceived as normal, and normal weight may be perceived as too thin or unhealthy. Some people still believe that chubby babies are the healthiest ones. And feeding behavior is strongly linked to love and security in almost all cultures.

The first step in breaking the hold of cultural norms and values is to become more aware of how they influence your thinking and your behavior. Then develop strong counterarguments and appropriate self-talk to refute them, at least within yourself if not with others.

Certain groups to which you belong may have unspoken norms for acceptable behavior that can influence your eating. Tom belonged to a men's club that had a regular, monthly lunch meeting. At one of these meetings, the menu called for beef stroganoff, but Tom, who had recently begun a serious weight management effort, called ahead and ordered a special diet plate.

At the meeting, the other men teased Tom about being on a diet. He did his best not to take the teasing seriously and just laughed off their gibes. He was prepared for this kind of reaction from his colleagues, and he kept mentally reminding himself that he was doing what was best for him (and that quite a few club members would do well to follow his lead).

Coping With Resistance to Authority

Connie joined a weight reduction program, but she resisted keeping records and doing the other assignments designed to help her be successful. She admitted that she had a running resistance to symbols of authority, and she chose to see record keeping and homework as just such symbols. This unfortunate perception kept her from losing weight, and she eventually dropped out of the program.

Sometimes other people are symbols of authority that bring up emotionally-charged memories, to which you react negatively. The message that you are not okay, or the possibility that you are not measuring up to the other person's standards, or the feeling of having no choice in the matter, can get your back—and your resistance—up.

If you instinctively react negatively to another's pressure on you to change, you are just as much influenced by that person, albeit in the other direction, as you would be if you complied with the other person's desires. Digging in your heels and resisting change, just because someone else wants you to change, often makes you a double loser—you retain unhealthy habits, and you feel angry and let down.

One way to counter this problem is to recall the benefits and costs you identified earlier that you associated with managing weight. Decide on your course of action based on this sort of analysis, not on your emotional reaction to someone else or to symbols that you allow to have power over your well-being.

When you find yourself resisting because someone is putting pressure on you, try discussing the situation and your feelings with that person. Are you being pressured because the other person feels it's for your own good, or because they believe that their own happiness depends on your changing to suit them? Often the answer to this question will affect your response.

Having clarified this, tell the other person how you are reacting to his pressure, and how you want him to behave instead. When people apply pressure on someone else to change, they seldom realize that their efforts are working in exactly the opposite direction.

Keeping Up Further Effort

Likewise, having actually gotten to goal weight, you may bridle at having to continue counting calories and watching what you eat. You may resist continuing in a maintenance program, telling yourself you know all you need to know and that you can make it on your own without further group support. Or you may be just plain tired of all the effort.

Reaching goal weight is exactly the time you should *not* terminate further support. Even though you now look slimmer and feel better about yourself, your new eating and exercise habits are not yet fully established. You are likely to be vulnerable to the lure of old ways. Continuing in a maintenance program is very important. One of the factors that characterizes those who succeed long-term is that they keep up the efforts that have brought success to date.

When Others Feel Threatened

Sometimes others feel threatened by your success. A person you care about may not want you to be slimmer—even if he claims he does. He or she may see your new-found slenderness as a threat to the relationship with you—if you look more attractive, you might not want that person any more, or someone else may steal you away.

Both Don and Joan were overweight. When Joan started losing weight, Don, who was not trying to lose weight, got upset. He kept insisting that she looked just fine to him. In fact, Don's real concern was whether he would continue to look fine in Joan's eyes, or that Joan might look good to someone else.

Finally, Don and Joan were able to communicate openly and honestly about their individual fears and needs, and to face the issues involved. Joan was able to reassure Don of her love and her commitment, regardless of his weight. As a result of the confrontation, Don began the difficult and long-delayed exploration of his own problems with self-esteem.

Sometimes resistance on the part of another to your weight management efforts can stem from fears on the part of the other person that he or she may lose influence or power over you if you reach and maintain a lower weight. Your success in losing weight may seem to signal a renegotiation of the rules of the relationship.

Frank used his wife's weight problem as an excuse to do what he pleased—stay out late, spend more money than they could afford on nonessentials, and generally indulge himself. When she complained, he brought up the subject of her weight. When she said nothing in the face of his indiscretions, he ignored her weight.

When she joined a weight management program and started losing weight successfully, Frank's ability to do as he pleased became threatened. First he tried to sabotage his wife by bringing her gifts of candy and sweets. When that didn't work, he became sullen and angry. The unspoken rules of their relationship were being threatened.

Unfortunately, many relationships that have these dynamics break up when one of the partners succeeds in losing weight. Usually such relationships were relatively unhealthy to begin with, and losing weight merely brought the problems into the open. Attempting to talk over the situation may help, but often such relationships can only benefit from professional help.

Once you reach goal weight, you may discover that your relationship needs to change as well. You may need to find new ways to relate to each other and to handle problems.

Often it turns out that getting to goal weight doesn't solve old problems. Rather, it can bring them to the foreground, and can produce some new ones.

Don't be afraid to reach out for help if you need it. Chapter 11 gives suggestions for getting professional assistance when new and potentially overwhelming problems emerge.

When You Get in Your Own Way

Occasionally weight management efforts are sabotaged by your own hidden agenda—to get sympathy or attention from others for having a problem with weight. This makes successful weight management almost impossible, because you get valuable payoffs for not losing weight, or for regaining weight lost, while appearing to be trying to overcome the problem.

As a child, Anna successfully got more attention from her mother than either her sister or brother because she was overweight. While her mother took her from doctor to doctor and worried about her eating behavior, Anna's father alternated between being angry over the doctors' bills and relieving his guilt for being angry by giving Anna gifts to make up for his reactions.

Anna's weight problem persisted until she got old enough to marry, at which time she reduced to normal weight long enough to snare a husband. Promptly after marrying, she regained weight and began repeating the same pattern of manipulation with her husband that she had used earlier with her parents.

In fact, Anna was quite unhappy with her life, even though she got certain benefits from having a weight problem. Her self-esteem suffered greatly, and she was constantly plagued with depression. She needed professional help, and her whole family needed to be involved. The only way Anna was able to get this help was to recognize that having a weight problem held certain payoffs for her, and that to break this cycle, she needed to learn new ways to relate to others and to create rewards for herself.

Likewise, when you are involved in attempts to manipulate other people, or to set them up to take the blame for your behavior (as Elsie did when she asked her husband to play watchdog at the party), or when you have a hidden agenda (like Betty had with her friend), you need to recognize that you are the problem—not them. Self-sabotage, not social influences per se, are affecting your eating behavior. Acknowledging that you are the problem is the first step toward being able to deal more effectively with it.

Circumstantial Pressure

Circumstantial social pressures come from the social situation, rather than from the influence of specific people. Such pressures may come from merely seeing food or observing others eating, from seeing advertising about food or eating, or from the social norms of the situation and the rules about socially appropriate behavior for the occasion.

Wanting to eat because you see someone else eating certainly seems like a social influence over which you have little or no control. In fact, how this affects you depends largely on how you allow yourself to think and react to seeing others eat. It is "natural" for the sight of food or of others eating to trigger vivid memories of past satisfaction from eating. But by allowing yourself to linger with these memories and mental images, you can actually provoke your body to salivate in preparation to eat. And once you begin to have such physical symptoms, together with thoughts and images about food, it is difficult to resist following through with eating.

One recourse is to turn your attention immediately to something else that does not involve food or eating. Another alternative is to purposefully remind yourself that you, and not the food you are seeing, are in charge of your behavior.

Use appropriate self-talk that will help you cope with the situation. For example, "Well, that may look good, but I just ate two hours ago and I'll be eating my regular meal in about an hour and a half. I'm not really hungry, and I'm not going to let my psychological appetite take over. I can observe this and still stay in control. I just need to remember how well I've been doing with my weight management so far."

In much the same way, you can use your self-talk to silently (or out-loud) combat advertising aimed at promoting eating. Or you can simply turn your attention to something else, and not allow yourself to think anymore about the advertisement. Learn to censor such information and remove it from your consciousness by refocusing on your commitment to your own health.

Parties and celebrations which involve food are another source of circumstantial social pressure—seeing others eating, or having to deal with the influence to eat that comes from the social norms of the situation. If you hang onto the thought that you just "can't resist" food that is available, inevitably you won't be able to resist it.

On the other hand, you can use tried-and-true behavioral techniques. You can be sure not to have tempting food in the house or otherwise available. When you are going to a party, eat before going and stay away from the hors d'oeuvres table. Finally, be prepared with appropriate self-talk.

Allow yourself to join in the celebrations, and keep reminding yourself that you choose food in moderation, that you are in charge of the food and it is not in charge of you. Be prepared with self-talk that will work for you, and practice in your imagination coping successfully with the situation.

Usually it takes a combination of being prepared with appropriate self-talk, having used mental rehearsal to imagine how you will act, and exerting environmental planning and control to cope most effectively with social influences. Sally played bridge regularly with her friends, and it was a matter of course for the hostess to have snacks placed on two corners of the bridge table during the game and to serve dessert afterwards. At first, Sally tried removing the snacks from the table corners, but the hostess repeatedly put them back.

Finally she spoke up and asked that the snacks be placed on the corners that were out of her reach. But when she spent an evening getting bad cards, her resolve to avoid inappropriate eating dissolved. She had to take stronger action.

The next time she called ahead to the hostess with some suggestions about a healthy dessert. Then she planned how she would bring her own snacks. She used imagery to see herself succeeding (even with bad cards). She came to her next bridge party prepared with appropriate self-talk, her own snacks—carrot and celery sticks, and her own diet drinks.

At first, the other bridge players were aghast. Carrot and celery sticks didn't seem like very exciting fare. But eventually they came around, and it became the norm for everyone to have healthy snacks and a healthy dessert on bridge nights.

Responding to "Put-Downs"

"Such a pretty face . . . what a shame."

"How could you let yourself go like that?"

"Oh, you are so thin, dear. You just don't look healthy."

And off you go to the nearest ice cream shop to nurse your wounded feelings. When a put-down comes from a friend or someone who supposedly cares about you, it is often hard to know how to respond. Usually they have no intention of hurting you. They may naively think it will motivate you to appropriate action, or they may simply be insensitive to the impact their remarks are having on you.

Your best response to a friend who puts you down is to communicate your feelings assertively, rather than aggressively. For example, "I'm sure you don't realize how your remarks are hurting me. I feel bad enough about my weight, and I have been making considerable effort to change it. What I'd like most from you is your understanding and support. If you want to help, please notice the progress I'm making and comment on that."

Or, "I've worked hard to reach goal weight. It may be a shock to you that I don't look like I used to. Please understand that I prefer to be thinner, and I'm sure you'll get used to my new look with time. In the meantime, I would prefer that you not mention to me any reservations you may have about my new appearance."

Unfortunately, however, some people you care about may use comments about your weight to hurt you and keep you down. Making put-downs may give them a sense of power over you. The key to coping effectively with this kind of situation is not to take it personally, even though the other person may intend it that way. Try using humor or your imagination to get some distance between yourself and the other person's aggression.

One woman whose husband seemed to enjoy putting her down about her weight used two strategies to cope. Sometimes she would co-opt his position—when he said something nasty about her, she responded with something totally outrageous and silly about herself. When he called her a "tub of lard," she responded, "Heavens, yes. I bet if I sat on you I'd smother you to death. You better watch out; I might do that some day." When her husband got this silly (and covertly threatening) statement instead of the usual sulking response that he was looking for, it would bring him to an abrupt halt.

At other times, she didn't feel like playing this game, and when he started in on her, she retreated inside her head and imagined seeing her husband before her making his usual put-downs, but now wearing diapers or dressed as a clown. She let his remarks fall on deaf ears because, after all, it was just an infant or a clown making them.

Likewise, you can create a mental picture of the person who remarks that you are too thin, imagining her sitting at a table stuffing herself, and mentally note that she isn't so slim herself. No wonder she wants to drag others to her level.

In a similar way, put-downs from strangers can be met with humor, retort, mental imagery, or deaf ears. One woman, who had been on the receiving end of a put-down from someone she didn't know, shot back, "Thank goodness you're not in the diplomatic corps." Alternatively, reply (with wide-eyed innocence), "Thank you for calling my attention to my weight; I hadn't noticed."

Fortunately, strangers don't generally make put-downs to those who are now slimmer. But because you aren't used to hearing compliments about your weight, you may misinterpret a remark as a put-down when it isn't. Judy was with a group of friends when a person who was stranger to her but a friend to the others joined the group. When the woman was introduced to Judy, she said, "Oh, you are so petite." Judy never thought of herself as "petite," and it was a shock. At first Judy thought the stranger was giving her a put-down. Then she realized that the compliment was real, and that she just wasn't used to thinking of herself as a thin person.

In all cases when you are the target of an actual put-down, take a deep breath and remember that it is really more a statement about the smallness and narrow-mindedness of the other person, than a statement about you. People tend to show prejudice and lash out at things that threaten them in some way. In all likelihood, the person making the put-down has some concerns about his or her own acceptability. She may have very low self-esteem, and putting you down is a way of building herself up. If you are able to conjure up a little sympathy for her, rather than allowing yourself to feel hurt or guilty, all the better.

Coping With Family, Friends, and Others

Family members, friends, co-workers, acquaintances and other people with whom you come in regular contact are collectively called your "social network." Whenever one member of the social network changes, it affects others to one degree or another. Change, even change for the good, can be disruptive and stressful. You need to anticipate and plan for this.

1.   *Talk it over.* Family and friends often resist your attempts to change because they must adjust in some way to the change. As part of her weight management program, Carmen started making some low-fat substitutions and reducing the amount of salt she used in cooking. She did not mention the changes she was making, and the family was not prepared for the changes in taste when she started cooking differently. Their objections, combined with Carmen's own beliefs that her family's needs and preferences came first, caused Carmen to go back to cooking a high-fat diet. If she had discussed her problem and the need to make changes with her family first, and asked for their understanding and support, the chances for successful change would have been better.

Explain to others what you want to do, why it is important to you, how you think it will affect them, and what you need from them in order to succeed. Be specific about what you want or need from others. Ask what you can do to make it easier for them, and invite them to talk to you if and when they experience any difficulties.

Then be ready to hear them out if they have problems or complaints. Don't dismiss their concerns as "silly" or "wrong." Look for a compromise solution that responds to at least some of the needs of everyone.

This strategy works well with co-workers too. Office parties and celebrations can be the undoing of the best weight management efforts. When others bring food in and make it available for the taking, or when birthdays are celebrated with a birthday cake or going out for a big lunch, speak up. Ask others not to offer food to you, and to put it in a place where you are less likely to be tempted. Agree to go to lunch only if the destination is a restaurant where you can order something healthy. Make these announcements before you are confronted with a temptation or difficult situation.

2.   *Take steps to reassure others.* Sometimes others feel threatened by change, as if it were a challenge for them, too, to change. When one person changes, others may become unsure about what this means. Joan needed to reassure Don that her losing weight did not change her commitment to their relationship.

Often change signals a shift in the balance of power in a relationship, or a change in the rules. Frank and his wife had to stop and take stock of their relationship, and find new, healthier ways of relating to each other. Taking care to reassure others and to say exactly what you need them to do to assist you can be very important for weight management success.

3. *Be specific about what you want.* Be specific about what you want others to do to support you. If you are trying to eat less, you might ask others to avoid leaving food in sight and to compliment your progress in making appropriate food choices. On the other hand, if others are paying too much attention to your weight management efforts, ask them to ignore them, or at least not mention them so often. Decide what assistance you need and then ask for it.

If you don't indicate what you need from others, they are unlikely to provide it. The burden to know what you need, and to ask for it effectively rests with you. Be assertive. Use the "DESC" approach:[1]

Describe what the person is doing or not doing that you don't like,

Express how you feel about it objectively and without blaming,

Specify what you want the person to do instead,

and finally spell out the

Consequences, especially the desirable ones, of such a change.

For example, suppose your son, John, munches potato chips in front of the television and this tempts you to eat too. You could begin to cope with this situation by describing the situation as you see it, pointing out gently the effects of his behavior, and then asking for his help and cooperation.

The interchange might sound something like this:

"John, I noticed that you eat potato chips while we're watching television. When I see you eating chips, it's really difficult for me to resist the temptation to eat some too. As I think you know, I've been pretty successful so far in managing my weight, and I don't want to backslide. I would be grateful if you would help me by not eating in front of me. Perhaps you could save your snacking for the kitchen and do it when commercials come on, or perhaps you could watch TV in your room if you really want to snack while watching TV. If you could do that for me, I'd really appreciate it."

Sometimes, however, others are all too ready to help. They seem to be looking over your shoulder every moment, noticing what you are eating and clucking their tongues.

When someone is paying too much attention to your weight management efforts, choose a neutral time (not when you have just turned around and found them watching you again), and try the DESC approach. Tell them what you observe about their behavior, how it is affecting you, and what you would prefer they do instead to support your efforts. Don't forget to tell them how grateful you will be for their help.

Although one woman actually felt like telling her daughter, who seemed to be shadowing her every move, to go soak her head, instead she said, "Dear, I appreciate your concern, but when I feel that I am being watched so closely, I feel even more like eating inappropriately. What would help me the most is for you to relax and not get on my case. Instead of noticing what I do wrong, notice what I'm doing right—but don't overdo that either. I think I'd do better with less attention, and I'd certainly feel more trusted by you."

4.   *Get others involved.* Other people are usually affected when you change in some way. In the example mentioned earlier of Colleen and Carl, when Colleen went on a diet, Carl no longer got to enjoy her company at the dinner table, because she was eating differently than he was. He found himself having only diet food to eat, unless he wanted to fix his own. He enjoyed going out to nice restaurants for dinner, but when she was dieting, Colleen didn't want to go. As Colleen's dieting continued, she became more irritable, which made Carl's life more stressful. To "make her feel better," he would bring home a box of candy or some sweets. He told himself that things would get back to normal when Colleen went off her diet.

The first thing Colleen needed to do to increase her chances of success was to discuss the problem with Carl, and get him involved in finding the solution. When Colleen simply announced that she was going on a diet, Carl felt this decision had been imposed on him. When he wasn't part of the solution, he became part of the problem.

When others are not concerned about their weight but are affected by your change efforts, get them involved in finding and implementing a solution. Avoid simply imposing your solution on them, or you may find them sabotaging your efforts.

5.   *Give a coherent message.* Sometimes we inadvertently encourage others to sabotage our change efforts by the way we communicate. Carmen probably betrayed her own doubts about the taste of food cooked the new way, and this encouraged the resistance of her family. Colleen's conflict over whether to eat "normally" or stick to her diet no doubt was communicated nonverbally, and influenced Carl to bring her candy and sweets.

Avoid saying "no" with your voice, but "yes" with your eyes. To avoid giving mixed messages, you must be clear within yourself about your commitment to achieving and maintaining a lower body weight. If you have secret doubts or hesitations, your nonverbal behavior—your tone of voice, body posture, or other physical behaviors—will betray this. Conflicting verbal and nonverbal messages invite others to decide for themselves what you mean, and often they interpret this in their best interests, not yours.

6.   *Learn to refuse without offending.* Once you are clear that you have the right to refuse, you need to be clear about your own preferences and needs. If you aren't sure what they are, take your time responding to requests.

When Sylvia's friend wanted to take her out to dinner to celebrate her birthday, Sylvia replied, "Thank you for the wonderful offer, but let me give it some thought. You know I've been working on managing my weight, and I'm not sure I'm ready to handle eating out in a restaurant just yet. May I let you know tomorrow?" Having negotiated some time to decide, Sylvia was able to sort through the pressures she felt to say yes, and evaluate whether accepting the offer was in her best interests.

Refusing someone, especially someone you care about, is often quite difficult. Wanting to be polite, wanting the other person's approval of you, or feeling sorry for the other person, may pressure you to agree, even if you don't really want to do so. Sometimes you may say yes initially, and then find an excuse to back down later. Generally this is a poor strategy that causes both you and the other person to feel bad.

The best approach once you are clear about what you want to do is to communicate clearly, directly, and objectively. It helps to acknowledge the other person and state your reasons for declining.

Sylvia decided it was not in her best interest at this time to confront eating in a restaurant. She said to her friend, "I've given your offer to go out to dinner for my birthday careful consideration, and I really want you to know how much I appreciate your thoughtfulness in inviting me. However, I really don't feel I'm ready to tackle eating out yet. How about going to a movie instead, or catching that new play in the city?"

7.   *Be ready to increase the level of assertion.* Sometimes telling a person "no," in your best clear, direct, and objective manner, still doesn't bring the desired results. You must be prepared to hold your ground and take a stronger stand. The woman trying to maintain goal weight who was being tempted by her friend at the pastry display case tried a "soft" refusal first, but when her friend persisted, she squared her shoulders and replied with conviction, "No, I won't!"

Another woman whose husband continued to bring her candy even after repeated requests that he not do so, was forced to move to a very high level of assertion to get results. When he once again brought her a block of solid chocolate, she thanked him for the gift, and as he watched, she carefully cut the chocolate into bite-size pieces and tossed it all down the kitchen disposal. He never brought her candy again.

Social Support Planning

Fill out the following information for each person in your social network who might be affected by, or be able to influence your behavior change effort.

Who	How They May Be Affected	How I Can Get Their Support

Specific Techniques for Getting Assistance From Others

Here are some techniques that can make it easier to get support from family and friends:

1.   *Plan to get support.* Identify those who may be affected by your weight management efforts and plan how you can get their support. Use the Social Support Planning form above to note who and how the people in your social network might be affected by your change efforts. Some strategies for getting their support might include assertively asking for specific assistance from them, reassuring them of your loyalty, or getting their cooperation in finding compromises.

2.   *Make a public commitment.* Having reached goal weight, you should write down the actions you intend to take to maintain goal weight. Write these down, both as a reminder to yourself and because having it in black and white often makes it seem more real. Post it in a public place, such as on the mirror or the refrigerator door, and tell your friends about your plan.

Contract

Sample

This is an agreement between (1) __Mary__
(person changing)

and (2) __John__
(support person)

For the period of this contract, from __May 5__

to: __May 12__ , (1) __Mary__

will: __take only one helping of food__
__at the evening meal__
(specify behavior)

To support (1) __Mary__ 's efforts, (2) __John__

will: __do the dishes for that meal__

(specify reward)

If (1) __Mary__ does not perform the specified behavior,

he/she will: __do the dishes for that meal and let__
__John choose which TV programs to watch__

Signed: (1) __Mary__

Signed: (2) __John__

Date: __May 1, 1992__

---

3. *Get a "buddy" to join in your effort.* Managing weight with a friend is a good motivator. Plan to get together at specific times to exercise, or go to support meetings together. Use each other as a resource for problem solving.

4. *Create a social contract.* This is a device, much like a regular business contract, that sets forth in a more formal way how one person will help another with weight management.

Suppose that Mary wants to limit her number of helpings at dinner to just one. She could make a contract with John covering a specified period of

---

Contract

This is an agreement between (1) _____
(person changing)

and (2) _____
(support person)

For the period of this contract, from _____

to: _____, (1) _____

will: _____

_____
(specify behavior)

To support (1) _____ 's efforts, (2)_____

will: _____

_____
(specify reward)

If (1) _____ does not perform the specified behavior,

he/she will: _____

_____

Signed: (1) _____

Signed: (2) _____

Date: _____

---

time for the commitment, and indicating what he will do and how she will be rewarded for succeeding. The contract also spells out the consequences if Mary does not meet her commitment. Such contracts can be a fun way to get others involved in your weight management efforts.

5. *Set up incentives and rewards.* Money is a wonderful motivator, but it isn't easy to give it to yourself. Instead, get the help of a friend. Decide what reward you will get for each new habit you want to establish. Then ask your friend to give you your rewards as you do what you have committed to do. For instance, you might want to earn $2 for each day you do your planned

exercise. Let your friend hold the money for you, and pay it back to you as you earn it.

It is important, however, to set it up so that there is a possibility of losing it, too. So instruct your friend to give you the reward only if you earn it within a certain time frame; otherwise, to give it to some person or group you would rather not support. (For example, if you are a Republican, you might tell your friend to send the money to the Democratic National Party if you fail to earn it back.) It is a good idea to be very specific about exactly what you will do, what the reward is to be, who is to get the reward if you don't, and the time period of the contract.

6.   *Join a class or program that relates to your needs.* There are many existing programs in the community that can augment your weight management efforts. The local YMCA usually offers low-cost, expertly-run health and fitness programs, as well as programs on stress management. Community colleges often offer courses on communicating more effectively.

Making a commitment to a program provides motivation and support from others who have made the same commitment. Often you can learn from others' efforts, and it helps to feel "I'm not alone in this." Dietitians often run support programs for weight management that are offered through a hospital, clinic, or recreation department. Check around for possibilities.

7.   *Get yourself involved in a meaningful project.* Finding a means of creating genuine satisfaction in your life will go a long way toward helping keep the weight off. Eating is often a source of self-nurturance and a means of relieving boredom. Getting involved in a career or commitment outside the home—something that will absorb your energy and give you pride and satisfaction from giving and creating—is an alternative to using food to fill the self-esteem gap.

Summary

Coping effectively with social influences involves balancing the inevitable influence of other people on your behavior, with what you know to be your best interests. You stand a good chance of getting the support of others for your weight management efforts if you challenge your old beliefs and assumptions, communicate more effectively, and take specific actions that will help you create social support.

References

1.   Bower, S.A., & Bower, G.H. (1976). *Asserting Yourself.* Reading, MA: Addison-Wesley.

Chapter 6

Improving Your Relationships

BEING ABLE to create and maintain satisfying relationships is a crucial factor in both the mental and physical health of all human beings. Through your relationship with another person, you come to know yourself better. Self-esteem builds on the reflection of yourself that you get from others. A positive self-image and a high level of self-worth are more likely when those around you hold you in high esteem and value you. Low self-esteem derives in part from being treated by others as if you were not important.

When the quality of a relationship is poor, estimates of self-worth and feelings of self-esteem usually fall. Sometimes the quality of the relationship is poor because one or both people involved have unresolvable problems. More often, it is because the people involved have certain beliefs or ways of thinking and behaving that impede a mutually satisfying relationship. They may simply lack certain relationship skills.

Although the subject of relationships is a broad one, healthy relationships are promoted when a person knows and accepts his or her individual rights and needs, is able to communicate these needs and rights in such a way as to get the needs met or protect the rights, and is able to effectively negotiate conflicting needs. Difficulty communicating assertively and managing conflict causes personal pain and jeopardizes relationships. Fortunately, it is possible to learn to improve your relationships, and doing so will increase your satisfaction of life, and ultimately make weight management easier.

Basics of a Healthy Relationship

Relationships are likely to be healthy and satisfying if they include four ingredients: intimacy, independence, respect, and cooperation.

98

Intimacy

Contrary to many people's beliefs, intimacy has little to do with sex. Intimacy in healthy relationships is characterized by a close relationship, involving mutual trust and liking. Building intimacy requires reaching out to and involving oneself with others, as well as disclosing the self appropriately to the other.

Some people have difficulty with intimacy. Those who are fearful of criticism or getting hurt tend to keep others at a distance. They do not trust others or dare risk disclosing their true selves.

Other people thwart the possibility of intimacy because they interpret the actions of others toward them as deliberately demeaning or threatening, even when there is little evidence for this. Still others prefer solitary activities over relationships with other people. Thus, fear, paranoia, and indifference are the enemies of intimacy.

Independence

In a healthy relationship, both parties experience themselves as independent. That is, they don't come to each other solely to have a need met; rather they *choose* to be with each other.

The person who has independence is assertive, expressive, spontaneous, loving, giving, vulnerable, open, trusting, playful, and accepting of self and others. She is not afraid to be alone, and periodically enjoys time to herself. Such a person feels her feelings, including anger and other unpleasant emotions, and uses these feelings appropriately. The independent person knows she is responsible for her own experience—her own emotions and behavior—but not for someone else's experience.

People who do not bring independence to a relationship are those who are always rescuing others, taking responsibility for other people's feelings and well-being, and trying to control outcomes that are beyond their control. Such people neglect their own needs and invalidate their own feelings and reactions.

Because they are emotionally, socially, and sometimes physically dependent on others and things outside the self, and because they neglect their own selves, such people have little self identity. Often they cannot make everyday decisions without excessive assurance or advice from others. They worry a great deal about other people, but neglect themselves. Sometimes they agree with others even when they know the other person is wrong, just to avoid the possibility of rejection.

Respect

A healthy relationship is also characterized by respect—for others as well as the self. The person who exhibits respect for others communicates honestly, accurately, and sensitively. She is specific and direct; she says what she means, and she means what she says. She is not afraid to ask for what she wants, rather than hoping the other person is able to read her mind. She doesn't drag up stuff from the past or catastrophize about the future. She tells the truth appropriately—i.e., when it is needed, when it can be heard by the other person, and when it is a fair representation of the whole truth.

The person who exhibits respect avoids blaming and is accountable for the role she played in an outcome. She listens to the other person and is open to feedback, but does not assume all of it necessarily applies to her. She can be empathetic to others, without taking on responsibility for their burdens. The respectful person avoids manipulating others or taking advantage of them. She acknowledges others and looks for the good in them.

Still, she is willing to confront unpleasantness and use her anger appropriately. She is willing to negotiate conflicting needs with fairness.

People who are not respectful of others are those who are aggressive or physically harmful to others, who lie, con, manipulate, or attempt to exploit others. Such people are often envious of others, and feel entitled to special treatment, or to exemption from the rules that others must follow. Often they try to be the center of attention, but lack the ability to anticipate how others may feel or react to their behavior.

Cooperation

Cooperation involves joint work toward a common end or purpose. Cooperation is usually needed to create fulfillment and satisfaction in life. To have cooperation requires accepting the self and others as imperfect beings (and not trying to change each other), being willing to work together and learn, being sensitive to each other's feelings (without being responsible for them), helping each other, and being willing to communicate openly, honestly, and assertively.

People who cooperate develop a shared vision that helps them resolve conflict. When they negotiate, they look for win/win situations, so that both sides get something of what they want. They give each other their due, and dispense liberal pats on the back. They listen without interruption, knowing they will have their chance to respond and be heard. When they commit to something, they do it, or they don't commit.

Cooperation is not fostered by people who insist they know what is right and refuse to listen to others' thoughts or opinions. Such people unreasonably insist that others submit to their way of doing things, and are reluctant to allow others to do things because they are convinced they will not do them correctly. They often resent suggestions of ways they could be more productive. Uncooperative people may criticize people in positions of authority, engage in scornful gossip, or protest what they feel are unreasonable demands made on them.

Healthy, satisfying relationships are possible. Fortunately, one person acting alone to be more intimate, independent, respectful, and cooperative is enough to bring about changes in others, that in time sow the seeds of better interpersonal relations. There is much you can do to improve your relationships.

Building Intimacy

True intimacy involves sharing your most inward self with another, revealing your private and personal feelings, and disclosing information about yourself—letting someone else know the good news and the not-so-good news about you. As a result you make yourself vulnerable to rejection or disapproval. But the paradox is that in the process of self-disclosure, you gain knowledge about your own values, needs, and feelings, and you make it safer for the other person to share himself with you. Only in that way can a close, intimate relationship develop.

There is an old saying: "oneness before twoness." It means that you need to become more comfortable with yourself, and more self-accepting, before you can become truly intimate with another. If you think there's no good news, or you discount or minimize the good news there is, or if the not-so-good news keeps you paralyzed from acting, you need to reexamine your beliefs and ways of thinking about yourself. You need to stop being so self-critical, and become more accepting and forgiving of yourself.

And, you need to be willing to accept both the good and the not-so-good news about someone else. By doing so, you allow the development of mutual trust and true intimacy. False intimacy and superficial relationships are created when one or both parties tries to maintain an image that they want the other person to see, rather than reveal their true selves.

Maintaining an image requires keeping certain information hidden, and this is a tremendous energy drain. As a result there is less energy left to go into the relationship itself. Sometimes a person is so caught up in his or her image that she is no longer in touch with who she truly is. Oneness before twoness. Know and accept yourself first. Then and only then is it possible to create a truly intimate relationship.

Assessing Your Willingness to Self-Disclose

How willing you are to share yourself with another will vary, depending on who else is involved and what aspect of yourself is a candidate for disclosure.

Choose three people who are significant in your life, but with whom you feel varying degrees of closeness. (For example, choose one person with whom you feel very close and comfortable, and another from whom you feel somewhat distant.) Write each of their names in the spaces provided in the self-test on page 103. Then rate your level of disclosure with each of them for each of the various aspects of yourself listed.

Now review your ratings on this self-test, notice which aspects are easier for you to talk about with which people. The more 3s you have, the more willing you are to self-disclose.

There are many blocks to self-disclosure—including fear of rejection, fear of punishment, fear of being laughed at, fear of being misunderstood, fear that someone will try to take advantage of you. Ask yourself what keeps you from self-disclosure about certain aspects of yourself with certain people. Decide whether you should try to improve your willingness to self-disclose.

How to Improve Your Self-Disclosure

The key to effective self-disclosure is balance—learning when to tell what to whom.[1] Revealing too little of yourself causes you to be perceived by others as withdrawn, closed, secretive, or out of reach, and that reduces your chances of developing more intimate, satisfying relationships. On the other hand, revealing too much of yourself too soon can make others feel uncomfortable.

In the first stages of a relationship, it is appropriate to reveal facts about yourself—what you do, where you live, where you went to school, and so forth. This is the first level of self-disclosure.

After both of you have revealed some facts and you are feeling more comfortable, you can proceed to the second level of self-disclosure—discussing "safe" thoughts, feelings, and needs. For example, you might talk about your tastes in music, your ambitions at work, things you want or are looking forward to in the future. (Generally thoughts, feelings, and needs, either from the past or related to the future, are safer than those rooted in the here-and-now.)

Eventually after you have both shared on this level enough to feel safe with each other, you can move to the third and final level of self-disclosure—taking the risk of telling the other person what you are thinking, feeling, and needing right now. You may show your emotions or reveal something you generally keep hidden. By doing so, you invite the other person also to share his current experience.

Self-Test 6.1

Self-Disclosure Assessment

Rating   0—I disclose *little or nothing* about this aspect.
1—I *lie* or *misrepresent* myself on this aspect.
2—I *share general things* about this aspect.
3—I am *completely open* about this aspect.

	Person #1: Name	Person #2:	Person #3:
Tastes, Preferences, Interests			
Food	____	____	____
Music, Art	____	____	____
Activities	____	____	____
Friends	____	____	____
Books, Movies	____	____	____
Attitudes & Opinions			
Politics	____	____	____
Religion	____	____	____
Morals	____	____	____
Personal values	____	____	____
Life philosophy	____	____	____
Work			
My strong points	____	____	____
My weak points	____	____	____
My satisfactions	____	____	____
My dissatisfactions	____	____	____
Money			
My debts	____	____	____
My income	____	____	____
My savings, investments	____	____	____
My habits or use of money	____	____	____
Body			
What I like about myself	____	____	____
What I dislike about myself	____	____	____
Health problems	____	____	____
Health or fitness habits	____	____	____
Self			
Emotions and feelings	____	____	____
Sexual relationships	____	____	____
Sexual problems	____	____	____
Fears	____	____	____
Needs or desires	____	____	____

Don't try to rush self-disclosure or intimacy. Some people need more time than others to develop a level of trust that will allow them to move through the various levels of self-disclosure. You can encourage them, however, by being the first to reveal yourself at a new level. Just be sure not to move on to the next level of self-disclosure until you sense they feel comfortable at the present level.

Knowing with whom to begin or to continue self-disclosing can also be a problem. A good way to test whether another person is a "safe" person with whom to self-disclose, is to use the share-check-share technique.[2]

Share something of yourself with another person. Then check the person's response. If he or she doesn't seem to listen, or appears to be preoccupied with her own agenda, or if he judges you, or invalidates your feelings, or tries to give you advice, you may not wish to share more of yourself with that person. Also, if that person rejects you or betrays you by talking about you or your confidences to someone else, that person is probably not a safe person with whom to continue to self-disclose.

However, if that person listens, is supportive, can empathize with you, and accepts your feelings without trying to rush in and change them, then it may be safe to continue self-disclosing. As you become more comfortable and able to trust yourself and others, you will be able to disclose more of yourself, *and* you will discover that you have more to share.

To have a more intimate relationship, you must be willing to be vulnerable and share yourself with others. As an aid to practicing and becoming more comfortable with self-disclosure, it helps to improve your conversation skills.

The Art of Conversation

To be a good conversationalist, you not only need to use self-disclosure appropriately, you need to know how to ask questions and be a good listener. Asking open-ended questions, rather than questions that invite a simple "yes" or "no" answer, is important. Remember that people generally like to talk about themselves, so it usually works to ask questions that inquire about the other person without prying. For example, instead of asking, "Didn't you live in Branner Hall at school?" try, "How did you like living at Branner Hall at school?"

Listening effectively means more than just keeping your mouth shut while the other person is talking. It involves periodically restating what you think you heard said, asking for clarification when necessary, and letting the speaker know your reaction to what was said. Good body language—maintaining eye contact, leaning slightly forward, smiling, and nodding now and then—signals that you are listening.

As noted earlier, self-disclosure facilitates the development of intimacy. To be a good conversationalist, however, you do not have to reveal your deepest needs and secrets immediately. Initially you may only share certain information, such as describing your job, your last vacation, or some funny experience. Eventually, you may decide to deepen the contact by disclosing thoughts, feelings, or needs.

It also helps to know how to give and receive a compliment, use humor, and have some knowledge of current events. Some steps that Dr. Phil Zimbardo suggests for overcoming shyness and developing skill as a conversationalist are:[3]

1. *Learn to begin talking.* If you find you have a hard time talking to anyone, try the following suggestions. These give you practice in talking, protect your anonymity, and don't require you to carry on a lengthy conversation.

   - Call a local department store and check on the price of something.

   - Call the sports desk at the local newspaper and ask for the scores of the last hometown basketball, baseball, or football game.

   - Call the library and ask the reference librarian what the population of the United States is, or ask for some other information that interests you.

2. *Practice giving and accepting compliments.* Tell someone that you like what he or she is wearing or how they look. Compliment some ability she exhibits: "You grow beautiful flowers." Or some aspect of their personality: "I love the way you laugh." Notice their possessions: "What a terrific car."

   When receiving a compliment, keep looking at the person giving it, smile, and just say, "Thank you." Don't drop your eyes, and never discount a compliment by saying something like, "Oh it's nothing really." Try returning the compliment: "Thanks, I like yours, too."

3. *Collect things to talk about.* To have a good conversation, it helps to have something to say. The easiest way to do that is to keep yourself informed.

   - Read the newspapers or news magazines and watch TV news.

   - Delve into one or two political, cultural, or whatever topics and become knowledgeable about them.

   - Keep a journal of interesting stories you have heard from others or that you have read; briefly review them before going into a social situation.

   - Practice how to introduce one of your topics by speaking into a tape recorder and then playing it back to yourself.

4. *Learn how to start a conversation.* First choose someone who looks approachable. Someone who is smiling at you or who is alone or wandering around is a good candidate. Remember to smile when you first speak. Then introduce yourself: "Hello, my name is ___." Try giving a compliment next: "I like your dress." Or ask for information or help: "Do you know who that person over there is?" Be willing to disclose something about yourself: "I don't feel particularly comfortable at parties." Offer to help: "May I get you another drink?" Or if all else fails: "What do you think about this weather?"

5. *Keep a conversation going.* Once you've started a conversation, the easiest way to keep it going is to ask more questions. Generally people like to talk about themselves or their interests if someone else shows interest. Or introduce one of your stories or items of interest by asking a related question: "Have you heard about the local controversy over school funding?" Be sure to share your reactions and opinions.

6. *Listen attentively.* Be sure to give the person speaking to you your full attention. Look at him or her, not down at the floor or around the room. Give other signs that you are listening, by nodding your head or perhaps just saying, "uh, huh" or "yes." Lean forward, sit up, stand closer, smile, and so forth.

7. *Don't assume.* Don't make assumptions without checking them out. If the person you are talking to is looking around the room during the conversation, you might ask, "Are you looking for someone?"—rather than assuming they don't like you. If you aren't sure you understand what someone is saying, ask them to repeat or clarify. They are likely to be pleased that you are interested enough to want to understand.

8. *Close a conversation correctly.* There are nonverbal signs that signal the end of a conversation. Breaking eye contact, moving your body as if to leave, leaning forward, smiling, nodding, or offering a handshake are all indicators of termination. Be sure to conclude the conversation by agreeing with your conversation partner, or by reaching some resolution in your conversation. Then show your appreciation: "I really enjoyed talking to you." And finally, indicate you hope to have contact in the future: "Hope to talk to you again."

Do not expect that you will be successful in implementing all of these steps for becoming a good conversationalist the first time you try. But give yourself credit for whatever steps you do take successfully. As you gradually accumulate more and more "little successes," your confidence will grow, your conversation skills will improve, and over time your ability to have relationship-building conversations with others will improve. As you become better at making social contact and creating friendships, you will become less likely to experience loneliness, and less likely to use food to fill the void.

Take Steps to Build Friendships

Friendships are usually based on: being physically close; being involved in mutual activities; having similar attitudes, values, background, personality, and interests; and expressing mutual liking. Not everyone you meet will be a good candidate for friendship.

When you do meet someone who may be a possibility, indicate that you would like to see her again to get to know her better. Set up a time no more than a few days later to meet for coffee or to go for a walk. (Going to a movie may not be a good choice unless you do something beforehand or afterwards that will allow you to have time to talk.) Friendships are built by spending time with another person, getting to know them, and letting them get to know you.

Communicating Assertively

Assertive communication is knowing and standing up for your rights and the rights of others. It involves communicating in a way that gets your needs met, while at the same time preserving the rights of others, and being sensitive to their needs.

When you are communicating assertively, you express your wants, ideas, and feelings in direct and appropriate ways. You feel self-confident and good about yourself at the time and also later. Other people feel that you respect and value them. Communicating assertively means communicating in such a way that the other person is enabled to act.

In contrast, *aggressive* communication is attempting to overpower another person and achieve your desires without regard for the other's rights or needs. When communicating aggressively, you express your wants, ideas, and feelings at the expense of others. Usually the intent is to dominate or humiliate the other person.

When you are communicating aggressively, you usually feel self-righteous and superior. Later you may feel embarrassed about what you said. Other people often feel humiliated, hurt, or angry as a result of being talked to in an aggressive way. You may get what you want, but it is at the expense of others. As a result, they may feel justified at trying to "get even."

Passive communication is when you allow someone else to ride roughshod over your rights and needs. You do not express your wants, ideas, and feelings, or if you do, it is in a self-deprecating way. Passive communication is usually an attempt to please others, or to avoid conflict.

When this is your primary way of communicating, you are likely to experience anxiety and feel disappointed with yourself. Often you feel angry afterwards, either with yourself or the other person, or both. When you communicate passively, others are likely to feel irritated by you, guilty about their behavior, or even superior to you. Or they may come to ignore you and your feelings and take you for granted. As you continue not to get what you want and need, your anger builds up. You may vent this anger with passive/ aggressive behavior.

Passive/aggressive behavior is a fourth style of communication. When you communicate passive/aggressively, your aggression is not as obvious or direct. Using the analogy of guerrilla warfare—rather than engaging in a frontal attack, you say or do things that are "hit and run" instances of aggression. Thus, you may use verbal "barbs"—short, cutting remarks—to the person toward whom you feel upset, rather than addressing directly what the problem is.

Passive/aggressive behavior finds expression in little acts of sabotage— "unavoidably" missing a deadline that the other person needs to have met to do his job well or easily, not keeping an agreement you have made, or doing things you know will upset the other person—and not doing things that would help the relationship, like helping out with chores.

When you are being passive/aggressive, you may collect "withholds"— things the other person says or does that upset you but which you do not communicate about at the time. Later you may confront him or her with a long list of things he does or doesn't do that upset you. You bring out all the "withholds" from the past to use in the present argument. (Withholds are evident when an argument ends up being about something other than what it started about.)

Aggressive communication, passive communication, or passive/aggressive behavior generally undermine relationships and create unpleasant emotions. In contrast, assertive communication helps foster better relationships because it promotes equality and fairness. Everyone is more likely to get at least some needs met. Problems and the inevitable little upsets that are encountered in every relationship are handled quickly and appropriately; they don't fester into bigger problems. Each person feels more self-confident, as well as respected by the other.

Lack of Assertiveness and Weight Management

A person who has had a weight problem may resort to an outright aggressive style of communication because she feels vulnerable, unsafe, or powerless. This may be a reaction to many real or perceived hurts from others related to being overweight. Many obese people involved in the "fat is beautiful" movement tend to communicate aggressively on this issue, which is perhaps understandable in light of the discrimination and ridicule heaped upon the obese by society.

More often, however, the person who has had to deal with a weight problem also exhibits passive or passive/aggressive behavior. She tends to accommodate others excessively, or may withdraw to avoid unpleasant interpersonal problems, confrontation, tension, and conflict. She may fear displeasing others, hurting another's feelings, or causing herself to feel rejected in some way.

Sometimes she is living out someone else's script, rather than pursuing her own. She may not know what her own desires are, or if she does, she puts them aside to accommodate what someone else wants. Her own needs get stuffed down, often with food. When she does seek to make her needs a priority, she often fails to stick to them when challenged.

Sometimes the person who takes a more passive role is looking for a "hidden bargain"—hoping that others will notice her self-sacrificing behavior, and love or respect her more. Then, when all her sacrificing doesn't pay off, she may resort to passive/aggressive behavior, further reducing the quality of her relationships and triggering painful emotions that produce more overeating.

While acting nonassertively seems from her perspective to be the way to get benefits, she pays a big price. She fails to get her own needs met adequately. Her self-confidence and self-esteem sink, and she may have to deal with her own anger directed toward herself as well as toward others. This kind of passive, dependent behavior may come, at least in part, from just not knowing how to speak up and communicate assertively. Perhaps she never learned assertiveness skills.

Research evidence demonstrates that children learn to behave by observing how their parents behave. If a child's role model is a nonassertive parent, he or she is likely to adopt the same style of interaction; a nonassertive mother is likely to have a nonassertive daughter. Alternatively, adopting a passive style may be necessary for survival if one or both parents is aggressive or threatening.

Becoming more assertive when you identify with a nonassertive role model, or when acting assertively might bring reprisals from someone, can be particularly difficult, but not impossible. However, beliefs and ways of thinking must be changed, and new ways of acting must be learned and put into practice.

Using Assertive Communication Effectively

Even though you may have one preferred style of communicating (assertive, aggressive, passive, or passive/aggressive), there will be times when you may choose to use a different style. It would be unreasonable to expect that you will never communicate in an aggressive or in a passive fashion, even after you have learned how to communicate assertively. The key is to strive to be assertive most of the time in situations where being assertive is appropriate.

There will be times when it is more appropriate to use an aggressive or passive style. Sometimes meeting someone else's aggressive communication with your own aggressive communication can cause the other person to back down, especially if he is trying to bluff you or if he thinks he can push you around. In the face of real threat, however, it may be wiser to behave passively. Or when the other person is emotionally overreacting or acting aggressively, it may be better to wait for things to settle down before you try asserting your position.

A passive/aggressive style, however, almost never works to your advantage. It usually represents a misdirected attempt to regain some power over the situation, or to get the other person to change without your having to deal directly with the problem. Sometimes there is also an element of needing to express anger or hostility without having to take responsibility for doing so. When you find yourself tempted to act in this way, take several deep breaths, mentally examine what you really want to have happen, and choose the best way to go about getting it done.

Waiting for the right opportunity to be assertive is usually the best answer. Then choose the right level of "muscle"—the amount of insistence or strength you put into an assertive statement.

Usually a low level of muscle, that is, the level of a polite request, will suffice. If this doesn't work, try increasing your verbal and nonverbal intensity, and use language that is straight to the point and not sugar-coated with polite words. (It is at this level that most women falter because of the lesson learned early that "nice girls are always polite.") If you still don't get the results you want, spell out the consequences of failing to comply (e.g., you will seek the intervention of an authority figure, or remove privileges, etc.) Finally, be prepared to actually do what you say you will do if an appropriate response is not forthcoming.

To become more consistently assertive, you need first to discover when it is that you tend not to communicate assertively. Having identified such "low assertiveness situations," you can then take steps to become more assertive. For people who have had a weight problem, those situations are often related to food and eating, or to asserting personal rights and needs. Use the following self-test to assess your assertiveness in certain situations that could relate to weight management.

Self-Test 6.2

Weight Management Assertiveness

Instructions: Each of the items below gives four possible options for responding to the situation described in the item. Even though a particular option may not describe exactly what you would do, judge the options in terms of how close they are to how you might respond. As your frame of reference in answering these items, assume that you are involved in attempting to lose weight by limiting your calories, avoiding high-fat and high-sugar foods, and increasing your exercise.

Since it is unlikely that you always use the same style of response in a particular situation, you may allocate points among the options. Assume that you have 10 points for each of the four alternative answers depending on how likely you are to react in that way. The more points you give to a particular answer, the more you would be likely to behave in that way. You may allocate all 10 points to just one answer if you feel that answer is the way you would always or almost always behave; or you may allocate the 10 points in any manner you wish, to show the likelihood of your reacting in the various ways described. Avoid the temptation to allocate unwarranted points to the option you know you "should" choose. Note how one person allocated points in the "Example" given:

Example

When someone you know well but haven't seen in a long time encounters you and comments about your weight, "How could you let yourself go like that?" you would:

a. __0__ Tell them it's none of their @X?/&! business.

b. __3__ Say something to the effect that you know they mean well but you feel hurt by their comment, given that no one is more aware of the problem than you are.

c. __6__ Pretend their remark doesn't bother you.

d. __1__ Comment that it's a good thing they aren't in the diplomatic corps.

Be certain that your answers add up to 10.

1. When someone I care about brings me a gift of high-calorie food or fixes something high in calories especially for me to eat, I tend to::

a. _____ Scold them for sabotaging my weight management efforts.

b. _____ Thank them for their thoughtfulness and indicate that I don't wish to lose ground with my weight management efforts by accepting the gift.

c. _____ Say nothing and eat some but not all of it.

d. _____ Figure I just can't win and eat the whole thing.

(continued)

Self-Test 6.2

Weight Management Assertiveness (continued)

2. When someone I work with brings food to work and leaves it in my sight, I tend to:

   a. _____ Tell them in no uncertain terms that they ought to know better than to leave it where it will be tempting to me.

   b. _____ Ask them politely to please move it to another place where I won't have to see it and be tempted (or ask if I may put it out of sight).

   c. _____ Say nothing and do my best to resist.

   d. _____ Say nothing and resentfully throw it in the trash at the first opportunity.

3. When someone I care about fixes a drink containing alcohol or lots of calories for himself or herself and wants me to join him or her in having a drink too, I tend to:

   a. _____ Express my annoyance that he or she is making weight management more difficult.

   b. _____ Indicate that I'd like to join them but I prefer having a diet drink.

   c. _____ Say nothing and join them.

   d. _____ Join them and bring up some aspect of their behavior that's been bothering me (or find something else to complain about).

4. When someone I care about asks me out to dinner, I tend to:

   a. _____ Reply in a hostile manner to the effect that I'm on a diet and can't go out to dinner.

   b. _____ Accept, if we can choose a restaurant that will make it easier for me to maintain my weight management progress.

   c. _____ Pretend to be delighted to go, and not let on about my weight management concerns.

   d. _____ Find an excuse why I can't go, and then feel deprived and upset with myself for being so fat.

5. When someone I care about eats tempting food in front of me, leaves tempting food out where I am likely to find it, or brings tempting food into the house, I tend to:

Self-Test 6.2

Weight Management Assertiveness (continued)

    a. _____ Get angry and tell them how I feel about such sabotage.

    b. _____ Point out how this affects me and indicate how I'd prefer they behave to support me.

    c. _____ Say nothing and cope the best I can.

    d. _____ Secretly fume and resolve not to buy their favorite food the next time I go to the market.

6. When someone I care about knows I have an exercise class at a particular time (or that I plan to exercise then) but still tells me they need me to take them to some appointment they have, I tend to:

    a. _____ Show how upset I am by telling them in no uncertain terms how selfish and thoughtless they are.

    b. _____ Hold firmly to my appointment, but help them think of another way they can get to their appointment.

    c. _____ Take them and figure I'll make it up next time.

    d. _____ Take them but give them the silent treatment.

7. When something happens that is unfair to me, or is an obvious error caused by someone else's carelessness, I tend to:

    a. _____ Get angry, tell them off, and get something to eat to feel better.

    b. _____ Examine the issue as logically and rationally as possible and try to work things out.

    c. _____ Resign to the situation as it is and feel helpless.

    d. _____ Ask who is their superior, implying that I am going to complain to that person.

8. When someone who is a friend, but not particularly close to me, wants to stop at a fast food restaurant for a bite, I tend to:

    a. _____ Tell them they ought to value their body more than to eat such high-fat, high-calorie food.

    b. _____ Indicate my preference for a place where I can get healthy food options.

    c. _____ Go along with their wishes.

    d. _____ Agree to their choice but criticize everything about the food, the location, the service, etc.

Scoring

After allocating 10 points for each of the 8 items, go back and add up your points for your "a" answers, for your "b" answers, and so forth.

Item:	"a" points	"b" points	"c" points	"d" points
1	_____	_____	_____	_____
2	_____	_____	_____	_____
3	_____	_____	_____	_____
4	_____	_____	_____	_____
5	_____	_____	_____	_____
6	_____	_____	_____	_____
7	_____	_____	_____	_____
8	_____	_____	_____	_____
Total Points	_____	_____	_____	_____
	Aggressive	*Assertive*	*Passive*	*Passive/ Aggressive*

Score Interpretation

Your total "a" points give you your aggressive communication score. Your total "b" points is your assertive communication score. Your total "c" points is your passive communication score, and your total "d" points is your total passive/aggressive communication score.

The highest possible score in any of these categories is 80. A "perfect" score would be to have 80 "b" points, indicating that you are always assertive in these weight management situations. The more likely case is that you will have a score of less than 80 in more than one type of communication. If your highest score is not your "b" score, you need to improve your skills in communicating assertively in situations that involve weight management.

Even if you have a higher "b" score than other scores, having more than 13 points in any of the other categories suggests there is some room for improvement in those areas.

Improving Your Weight Management Assertiveness

One of the most important assertiveness skills for successful weight management is the ability to say "no" and stick to it. Before you can begin to do this, you need to examine and challenge the self-defeating beliefs that make refusing difficult for you. You need to revise your assumptions about what making a refusal means, and you need to be prepared to cope with the possible reactions your refusal may produce.

Refusing someone's request does not mean that you are selfish. It means that at this particular time you cannot or will not accommodate this person's wants or needs. It means you recognize your own needs and limits, and judge that everyone will be better served by your refusing at this time.

Refusing does not mean that you don't really care for this person. It's true that caring involves doing some things for the other person, but caring does not mean limitless giving, and there are times when not giving is more appropriate.

Refusing does not mean that you are rude or impolite. This is the trap that catches many women, who have been trained all of their lives to be "nice." Refusing when you feel it is in your best interest to do so is healthy.

Refusing does not mean that you will never be asked again. You can reduce the likelihood of this by asking for a "rain check," or expressing your fear that he will not ask again at a time when you could accommodate.

Refusing does not necessarily mean that the other person will be hurt or offended, and if he is, this is his problem, not yours. It is better to endure some short-term discomfort from a negative reaction, than the long-term unpleasantness and accompanying resentment that agreeing to something you don't really want to agree to can bring.

Guidelines for Making a Refusal

1. *Be direct, instead of giving excuses.* An excuse may be a lie or it may be the truth, but it is a reason given to justify some action or behavior. Often, an excuse is invented or embellished so that one's conduct will be overlooked. When an excuse is given while attempting to make a refusal, it provides the other person with a pretext for arguing with your refusal. That is, they may attempt to persuade you to comply with their request by attacking your rationale. If possible, it is better not to provide such an opportunity. Just say "no."

2. *Tailor the refusal to the situation.* Sometimes it may be appropriate to give an explanation when you make a refusal. This is especially so when you are refusing a superior or someone who would react negatively without an explanation. In this case, the point of your explanation should be to communicate something personal about your situation and that you feel firm in making the refusal. Thus you might say, "Thank you but no; I don't eat chocolate." Such a refusal-with-explanation is less likely to invite counterarguments than, "Gee, I wish I could, but I'm trying to watch my weight."

When you have mixed feelings—part of you wants to say "yes" —be careful about sharing this. The other person may interpret this as an invitation to talk you out of your refusal.

Sometimes it may be necessary to acknowledge something about the other person in order to make the refusal stick. For example, "I appreciate that you worked really hard to make this special dessert. It looks really lovely. I hope you'll understand. I'm just not eating high-calorie desserts right now."

Alternatively, you may want to offer a compromise. "I can see you have gone to a lot of trouble to make such a lovely dessert. I'll just have a bite of my husband's portion, but I don't want a serving of my own, thank you."

3. *If necessary, change the situation.* When you find yourself repeatedly having to say "no" and feeling increasingly uncomfortable about it, you need to determine whether there is any way to restructure the situation so that the other person does not continue making the same request of you. For example, if each time you meet your friend for lunch, she asks you to share a dessert with her, the best solution may be to avoid going to lunch with her.

Many people who have had to deal with a weight problem tend to communicate passively, rather than assertively, perhaps because they lack skills or training in being assertive, or perhaps because they wish to avoid potential interpersonal conflict. This style of communicating can make successful weight management especially difficult, because one important assertive communication skill needed for success is to be able to say "no" and make it stick.

In addition to refusing assertively, the person most likely to be successful in maintaining goal weight is also better able to manage interpersonal conflict. The next section focuses specifically on conflict management skills.

Managing Interpersonal Conflict

Conflict arises for a variety of reasons: values differ, expectations are unrealistic, unwarranted assumptions are made, there is an apparent breach of fairness, judgments come into play, there are hidden agendas, agreements are not kept, role definitions lack clarity, someone makes a mistake or behaves inappropriately—to name just a few.

The essence of conflict is a difference of opinion or perspective. The hallmarks of most conflict situations are disagreement and opposition. Sometimes criticism, hostility, and aggression are also involved. Conflict is always disruptive, because it demands change.

Some conflicts can be positive and produce growth. Conflict can serve to clarify issues, initiate problem solving, stimulate negotiation, and ultimately deepen and strengthen relationships. Ideally, everyone can come out feeling that he or she has gained something as a result of the conflict.

Sometimes conflict is unnecessary and unwarranted. It tends to be destructive when someone ends up feeling he or she is the loser.

Communicating assertively may bring you into conflict with others, especially if they have been used to getting their own way and now you are changing the rules. Even in the best of relationships, there are times when one person does something that interferes with the other's wishes, needs, or actions.

A key to relating more satisfactorily with others is having the ability to handle the inevitable conflicts that come up. By communicating assertively, rather than aggressively or passively, you increase the chances that all parties in the conflict will feel heard and feel satisfied with the resolution.

Overweight and Interpersonal Conflicts

Conflict is always unpleasant, but it is especially so for those who have had to deal with a weight problem. They are more likely to take things personally. The low self-esteem they usually bring to a situation makes them more vulnerable to the emotional arousal inherent in interpersonal conflict.

Past experiences of criticism, rejection, and discrimination create anxiety, and conflict threatens more of the same. If the participants don't simply withdraw from the conflict, they are likely to "pull punches," or do things that are not natural for them, to avoid the risk of personal rejection.

Anger is repressed, and the more it is repressed from situation to situation, the more the pressure builds. Eventually repressed anger itself poses a threat in a situation of interpersonal conflict and confrontation, because the person trying to continue repressing it may fear losing control. A vicious cycle is set in motion—conflict brings fear of criticism and possible rejection, which threatens loss of control, producing repressed anger, leading to more conflict, and so on.

Managing Conflicts More Productively

The first step to managing conflict more productively involves developing a greater awareness of how you experience and respond to conflict. Learn to listen to yourself; notice what it is you say to yourself in the midst of a conflict situation. Acknowledge honestly your emotions; don't try to deny how you feel because of old tapes about how being angry isn't "nice."

Become more aware of your physical reactions in a conflict situation. Tune into your own nonverbal behaviors and the feedback you get from others; watch their nonverbal reactions to you—how they physically react in a conflict situation. Assess how you typically manage conflict, and whether changes need to be made.

Assessing Your Conflict Management Style

To help you better understand how you approach and handle conflict, complete the *Conflict Management Style Survey* self-test that follows.

Self-Test 6.3

Conflict Management Style Survey

Instructions: Choose a single frame of reference for answering all 15 items (e.g., work-related conflicts, family conflicts, or social conflicts) and keep that frame of reference in mind when answering the items.

Allocate 10 points among the four alternative answers given for each of the 15 items below.

Example

When the people I supervise become involved in a personal conflict, I usually:

a. __3__ Intervene to settle the dispute.

b. __6__ Call a meeting to talk over the problem.

c. __1__ Offer to help if I can.

d. __0__ Ignore the problem.

Be certain that your answers for each question add up to 10.

1. When someone *I care about* is actively hostile toward me, (i.e., yelling, threatening, abusive, etc.) I tend to:

   a. _____ Respond in a hostile manner.

   b. _____ Try to persuade the person to give up his/her actively hostile behavior.

   c. _____ Stay and listen as long as possible.

   d. _____ Walk away.

2. When someone *who is relatively unimportant to me* is actively hostile toward me, (i.e., yelling, threatening, abusive, etc.) I tend to:

   a. _____ Respond in a hostile manner.

   b. _____ Try to persuade the person to give up his/her actively hostile behavior.

   c. _____ Stay and listen as long as possible.

   d. _____ Walk away.

3. When I observe people in conflicts in which anger, threats, hostility, and strong opinions are present, I tend to:

   a. _____ Become involved and take a position.

   b. _____ Attempt to mediate.

   c. _____ Observe to see what happens.

   d. _____ Leave as quickly as possible.

Self-Test 6.3

Conflict Management Style Survey (continued)

4. When I perceive another person as meeting his/her needs at my expense, I am apt to:

    a. _____ Work to do anything I can to change that person.

    b. _____ Rely on persuasion and "facts" when attempting to have that person change.

    c. _____ Work hard at changing how I relate to that person.

    d. _____ Accept the situation as it is.

5. When involved in an interpersonal dispute, my general pattern is to:

    a. _____ Draw the other person into seeing the problem as I do.

    b. _____ Examine the issues between us as logically as possible.

    c. _____ Look hard for a workable compromise.

    d. _____ Let time take its course and let the problem work itself out.

6. The quality that I value the most in dealing with conflict would be:

    a. _____ Emotional strength and security.

    b. _____ Intelligence.

    c. _____ Love and openness.

    d. _____ Patience.

7. Following a serious altercation with someone *I care for deeply*, I:

    a. _____ Strongly desire to go back and settle things my way.

    b. _____ Want to go back and work it out—whatever give-and-take is necessary.

    c. _____ Worry about it a lot, but do not plan to initiate further contact.

    d. _____ Ask who is their superior, implying that I am going to complain to that person.

8. When I see a serious conflict developing between two people *I care about*, I tend to:

    a. _____ Express my disappointment that this had to happen.

    b. _____ Attempt to persuade them to resolve their differences.

    c. _____ Watch to see what develops.

    d. _____ Leave the scene.

continued

Self-Test 6.3

Conflict Management Style Survey (continued)

9. When I see a serious conflict developing between two people who *are relatively unimportant to me,* I tend to:

   a. _____ Express my disappointment that this had to happen.

   b. _____ Attempt to persuade them to resolve their differences.

   c. _____ Watch to see what develops.

   d. _____ Leave the scene.

10. The feedback that I receive from most people about how I behave when faced with conflict and opposition indicates that I:

    a. _____ Try hard to get my way.

    b. _____ Try to work out differences cooperatively.

    c. _____ Am easygoing and take a soft or conciliatory position.

    d. _____ Usually avoid the conflict.

11. When communicating with someone with whom I am having a serious conflict, I:

    a. _____ Try to overpower the other person with my speech.

    b. _____ Talk a little bit more than I listen.

    c. _____ Am an active listener (feeding back words and feelings).

    d. _____ Am a passive listener (agreeing and apologizing).

12. When involved in an unpleasant conflict, I:

    a. _____ Use humor with the other party.

    b. _____ Make an occasional quip or joke about the situation or the relationship.

    c. _____ Relate humor only to myself.

    d. _____ Suppress all attempts at humor.

13. When someone does something that irritates me (e.g., smokes in a nonsmoking area or crowds in line in front of me), my tendency in communicating with the offending person is to:

    a. _____ Insist that the person look me in the eye.

    b. _____ Look the person directly in the eye and maintain eye contact.

    c. _____ Maintain intermittent eye contact.

    d. _____ Avoid looking directly at the person.

Self-Test 6.3

Conflict Management Style Survey (continued)

14. When someone does something that irritates me (e.g., smokes in a nonsmoking area or crowds in line in front of me), my tendency in communicating with the offending person is to:

    a. _____ Use strong, direct language and tell the person to stop.

    b. _____ Try to persuade the person to stop.

    c. _____ Talk gently and tell the person what my feelings are.

    d. _____ Say and do nothing.

15. When someone does something that irritates me (e.g., smokes in a nonsmoking area or crowds in line in front of me), my tendency in communicating with the offending person is to:

    a. _____ Stand close and make physical contact.

    b. _____ Use my hands and body to illustrate my points.

    c. _____ Stand close to the person without touching him or her.

    d. _____ Stand back and keep my hands to myself.

Adapted from: J. William Pfeiffer and Leonard D. Goodstein, (Eds.), *The 1982 Annual for Facilitators, Trainers, and Consultants*, San Diego, CA, Pfeiffer & Company 1982. Used with permission.

Scoring

Instructions: When you have completed all 15 items, transfer your scores to the appropriate columns below, and add your scores for each column.

Question No.:	Column 1 "a" points	Column 2 "b" points	Column 3 "c" points	Column 4 "d" points
1	_____	_____	_____	_____
2	_____	_____	_____	_____
3	_____	_____	_____	_____
4	_____	_____	_____	_____
5	_____	_____	_____	_____
6	_____	_____	_____	_____
7	_____	_____	_____	_____
8	_____	_____	_____	_____
9	_____	_____	_____	_____
10	_____	_____	_____	_____
11	_____	_____	_____	_____
12	_____	_____	_____	_____
13	_____	_____	_____	_____
14	_____	_____	_____	_____
15	_____	_____	_____	_____
Total Points	_____	_____	_____	_____
	Aggressive/ Confrontive	*Assertive/ Persuasive*	*Observant/ Introspective*	*Avoiding/ Aggressive*

Score Interpretation

Aggressive/Confrontive

A high score indicates a tendency toward "taking the bull by the horns" and a strong need to control situations and/or people. Those who use this style are often directive and judgmental.

Assertive/Persuasive

A high score indicates a tendency to stand up for oneself without being pushy, a problem-solving approach to conflict, and a willingness to collaborate. People who use this style depend heavily on their verbal skills.

Observant/Introspective

A high score indicates a tendency to observe others and examine oneself analytically in response to conflict situations, as well as a need to adopt counseling and listening modes of behavior. Those who use this style are likely to be cooperative, even conciliatory.

Avoiding/Reactive

A high score indicates a tendency toward passivity or withdrawal in conflict situations and a need to avoid confrontation. Those who use this style are usually accepting and patient, often suppressing their strong feelings.

Now total your scores for Columns 1 and 2 ("a" total plus "b" total) and add these together to get your "A" Score. Total your scores for Columns 3 and 4 ("c" total plus "d" total) and add these to get your "B" Score.

Column 1 Score:_____ + Column 2 Score:_____ = _____"A" Score

Column 3 Score:_____ + Column 4 Score:_____ = _____"B" Score

Next, find the difference between these two scores by subtracting the smaller from the larger.

If your "A" Score is 25 points or more higher than your "B" Score, it may indicate a tendency toward a more aggressive/assertive conflict management style. You are not afraid to speak out, even to the point of becoming hostile, in response to conflict. If your "B" Score is 25 points or more higher than your "A" Score, you tend to take a more conciliatory, even passive approach, possibly withdrawing from or avoiding conflict as much as possible.

What insights have you gained about yourself and your reaction to conflict as a result of answering the questions in this survey? What changes, if any, do you need to undertake?

Coping With Criticism

Chapter 8, *Managing Anger and Loneliness*, deals specifically with coping with your own anger, and suggests techniques to use for this purpose. One important point made in that chapter that applies in conflict situations is to avoid taking things too personally. When you get negative feedback or criticism from another person, remember that often this is more a statement about that person than it is about you.

People tend to criticize others for the very things they dislike or fear the most in themselves. When you get negative feedback, try to hear it as objectively as possible, and not take it personally. Ask yourself what kernel of truth might be contained in the criticism and how you can profit from hearing it. Let the part that doesn't apply to you just go past you.

Feedback that is constructive can help you learn from your mistakes and improve your performance. Sometimes feedback is merely an unnecessary reminder of something you know you did wrong. In either case, it is better to merely acknowledge the feedback and avoid making excuses or giving explanations unless absolutely necessary.

At other times, criticism can be both nonconstructive and manipulative. Your critic may intend such statements as put-downs or aggressive confrontations. There are three ways to handle such criticism.

You can *agree in part* with your critic. Find some part of what the critic is saying that you can honestly agree with; acknowledge just that part and ignore the rest. If he exaggerates, using such words as "always" and "never," you may be able to rephrase the sentence with a more moderate word such as "sometimes." You could also agree that he sees the situation a particular way, without agreeing that the situation is actually that way. For example, "Yes, I can see how you might feel I spent too much money on that."

You can also *agree in probability* when there is some chance that your critic is right. For example, "It could well be . . ." or "You might be right . . ." You are not agreeing that he is right. Just that is it possible he could be right— or wrong.

Furthermore, you can *agree with the logic but not the assumption* your critic is making. Thus, when your mother scolds, "If you don't discipline those children, they'll grow up to be criminals," you can agree with the logic, even though you don't agree that you fail to discipline your children.

There is a difference, of course, between criticism—which may or may not be "constructive"—and put-downs or ridicule. When confronted with put-downs or ridicule, you should realize that the other person is being aggressive in order to win her point by bringing you down, intimidating you, or causing you to respond in kind. Generally such people are good with sarcasm and abusive expression, and responding in kind is merely playing the game their way—the way they are more likely to win.

The best way to handle this situation is to take a "martial arts" approach—flow with the blow. Don't let it get to you. Keep your calm. Stay centered. Reaffirm your point of view but don't let their verbal blows get to you. If you do find anger beginning to rise in you, take a deep breath and remind yourself to stay centered and balanced.

In some cases, you may not be able to tell whether the criticism is constructive or meant to be destructive. Or your critic's comments may appear to you to be "out-of-left-field." Don't hesitate to ask for clarification. When your critic uses global labels or generalizations such as, "You're not pulling your weight around here," ask for more information. "What am I doing or not doing that bothers you?" Pin him down to specifics.

Ask for a concrete example that shows what he means. This should enable you to get a clear understanding of the person's gripe, and be better able to respond. If his complaint is not clarified, it is likely that your critic is being manipulative and aggressive toward you.

Avoiding Conflict Situations

Ideally, the best approach is to head off the conditions that create a conflict situation. This usually means being willing to communicate openly and honestly about your needs, making sure that both parties understand and agree on what needs to be done and on the rules of the relationship, and being aware of the subtle cues that suggest when a problem may be brewing. Conflict can often be avoided by:

1. *Being sure to communicate up-front.* Sometimes a conflict situation is created by actions or omissions that happened long before the actual conflict. When one or both parties does not express their wants or needs early on, or assumes that the other knows what these wants or needs are, or pretends or rationalizes to herself that she "can live with" certain unacceptable conditions, the seeds of conflict are planted. When a person avoids confronting a problem when it first shows up, it is only a matter of time before the problem—and the potential for serious conflict—gets worse.

It is essential for the long-term health of a relationship (as well as of the people in the relationship) to be willing to talk about and reach agreement on important issues. The husband and wife who don't talk about how many children they want, until after they have had one and she wants another but he doesn't, create a potentially disastrous conflict situation. Similarly, two people who start a new business together, but don't get into the specifics of who is responsible for what, lay the groundwork for future conflict.

2. *Continuing to communicate.* Even if you do take care to discuss and plan for potential problems in the beginning, circumstances change, and people can change their minds. Continuing to communicate openly and honestly on an ongoing basis, even when it may be uncomfortable, is part of avoiding major conflict later.

Sometimes there is a misunderstanding on the part of one party about what was agreed. Negotiation and compromise are often easier when it happens earlier, before tempers flare. Discussing differences of opinion without blaming or rancor, and being willing to listen to the other's point of view helps a lot.

3. *Paying attention to warning signals.* "All of a sudden he just blew up. I was so surprised. I didn't realize our remarks were making him upset." This person wasn't paying attention to the warning signals.

There are almost always warning signals of problems and impending conflict. Often they are nonverbal signals sent out by the person getting upset—a tendency to become quiet and not engage in eye contact, tightness around the mouth and face, narrowing of the eyes, clipped verbal responses, a curt tone of voice, sighs, nostrils flaring, flushing of the face, and so forth.

When you begin to pick up warning signals, ask for clarification: "Are you upset about something?" Be willing to listen and actually hear what the other person is saying. Even if you feel that he is being irrational, remember that his emotions are aroused at the moment. You are more in control, so choose a conciliatory approach until he settles down. At another, more neutral time, you may wish to be more assertive in response to the circumstances prompting the anger.

Sometimes there are recurring situations that could benefit from an "early warning system." One example is that of the wife who didn't pay attention to the warning signals that her husband was getting upset by her remarks in a social situation. This happened with some frequency, and her ability to pick up her husband's cues tended to be reduced if she had a glass of wine or two.

They could have benefited from a forthright conversation at a neutral time to discuss the recurring problem, and to plan ahead for future ones. They needed to establish and agree upon a more direct but subtle signal that the husband could use in social situations to tell his wife he was becoming annoyed.

For example, the husband might say to the wife, "Gee, was that the telephone ringing?" This abrupt and out-of-left-field change in the conversation would be her signal to pay attention to what she was saying and change her remarks. With such an early warning system, they would have been better able to avoid similar future conflict.

4. *Assessing your conflict history.* Your experience with conflict and anger in the past has a direct impact on your reaction to and ability to manage conflict and anger now. Understanding this connection can sometimes help you manage your reactions today. The woman who has grown up in a home filled with conflict and anger, and who has developed a fear of that conflict and anger, understandably tries to avoid anger at all costs even today.

Yet running away from conflict, or always being conciliatory, may not be the best way to cope with conflict. It is important to develop a wider range of responses to conflict. Sometimes it is appropriate to be conciliatory. At other times it is appropriate to be assertive. In the face of some kinds of aggression, it may be wise to withdraw until a safer time. Rarely is it necessary to be aggressive, except possibly to ward off other aggression.

Another woman grew up in a home in which children were not allowed to have or express anger (but the parents were). She learned as a child to repress her anger, and this carried over into adulthood. As a result, it would periodically reach unmanageable proportions, and at some point explode into aggressive behavior.

At times, coming into conflict with someone would trigger a release of anger, and at other times she would repress it. Since she had never learned to express anger appropriately, her response to conflict would sometimes appear extremely hostile, often causing the other person in the conflict situation to withdraw. This woman had to learn to accept her anger, express it appropriately, manage her level of physical arousal, and pay attention to the cues that signaled danger ahead from potential conflict.

Confronting Anger in Others

Often the difficulty in a conflict situation comes from having to face someone else's anger. Most people regard anger as something that is "not nice" and should be avoided. But there are ways to make confrontation easier and to facilitate a better outcome:

1.   *Don't let yourself get hooked into someone else's anger.* Maintain your "cool" by using positive self-talk, avoiding taking things personally, and staying relaxed. If the other person knows your "hot buttons"—what will cause you to get emotionally involved in the conflict—he can predict your behavior, and he is likely to use this to gain power over you in a conflict situation.

2.   *Temporarily abandon your need to be logical.* Logic and reason won't dissolve fear or anger in others, and can even intensify their emotion. Applying reason in such a situation makes the other person feel irrational in expressing his emotions. Instead, listen and deal at the emotional level— provide comfort, understanding, and acknowledgement of the feelings being expressed.

3.   *Be willing to make conciliatory gestures.* You may be able to defuse the situation by agreeing or appearing to agree with the angry person. Find some part of what the angry person is asserting that you can honestly agree with, and acknowledge that she is right about that part. Then ignore the rest of what she is saying. For example, if you are accused of "always ignoring" her, you might be able to say, "Yes, when I'm watching the evening news, I do tend to get engrossed and not hear you."

4.   *Ignore verbal abuse.* Don't take it personally. This is just a ploy to gain power over you, and the only way it can work is if you let it. Remember that they are engaging in character assassination because of their own misery, and not necessarily because you are wrong or bad.

5.   *Avoid escalation.* Request that voices be kept at a normal tone and that verbal abuse be curtailed. If this request is not heeded within a reasonable time, signal the need for a "time out"—a preplanned period of time when all interaction is to stop temporarily while tempers settle. During this time both people should get out of each other's sight and engage in something that will soothe upset feelings.

Be sure that there is an established time to get back together, however. Otherwise, the person attempting to withdraw may be further confronted or even restrained by the angry person, who now regards this as a fighting strategy.

6.   *Resolve residual stress.* Once a conflict situation is past, remember that you are likely to have some residual arousal and emotions. You need to be prepared to deal with this. Do a relaxation exercise to let go of muscle tension, or go for a long walk. Don't dwell on the events of the conflict.

Try to clear and settle your mind. Take care of yourself. Remind yourself that conflict is something that you must learn to handle if you are to be successful in the long-run in managing your weight and your life. Consider what lessons you have learned, and how you can improve your conflict management skills in the future.

Coping With Potentially Violent Conflict

Unfortunately, there can be times when a conflict situation turns "ugly," and violence is a possibility. Instances of wife battering and other forms of physical abuse are becoming increasingly recognized. Some things you can do to cope include:

1.   *Learn to recognize the signs of potential violence.* The person who is most likely to become violent is one with a history of previous violence, one who has been using alcohol excessively or has been taking drugs, and one who exhibits certain telltale, nonverbal behavior such as taut muscles, clenched fists or jaw, flared nostrils, eyes bright and sometimes bloodshot, retracted lips, and either a flushed red face or a pale white face. If your gut feeling tells you there is danger, heed it.

2.   *Prepare yourself to cope.* Keep your calm; breathe deeply and slowly, and mentally coach yourself on what to do next. Look for a graceful or convenient exit or for possible sources of assistance. Do not block the other person's exit or attempt to restrain him if he wants to leave. Think of as many

options as you can to resolve the situation. No matter how offensive the language, don't let it get to you. Force yourself to be as detached as possible; this will give you an advantage.

3. *Try to de-escalate the situation.* Maintain a non-threatening body posture—arms at your side, palms open. Keep your voice calm and soothing, and don't touch the other person. Try to get him to move out into the open, as this sometimes has a calming effect. Don't try to problem solve or find explanations; just look, listen, and deal on the surface to try and de-escalate.

4. *Use distraction if possible.* Change the subject, ask an irrelevant question, or make an "off-the-wall" comment, such as, "I thought I heard a dog barking," to try and break the tension.

Coping With Losing

It is inevitable that sometimes you will feel as though you are the loser in a conflict situation. When that happens, the best you can do is to recover as well as possible. Using any of the variety of stress reduction techniques — progressive deep muscle relaxation, deep breathing, meditation, and vigorous physical exercise—will help.

Taking charge of your thinking is also essential for recovery. This may involve temporarily denying that something undesirable is happening, or finding ways to distract your attention to other concerns. You may have to suspend judgment and mentally distance yourself from the event, until you are finally able to accept it. Ultimately this may mean reprogramming your beliefs and way of thinking about the situation, or seeing it as a "learning opportunity." In any event, it is important to avoid dwelling on what is past, and to get on with living.

Summary

There is much you can do single-handedly to improve your relationships. First, you have to understand what it takes to have intimacy. This begins with appropriate self-disclosure. It also helps to know how to have casual and friendly conversations.

All relationships work best when you are able to communicate in such a way as to get your needs met while still respecting the needs of others. Usually, this means communicating assertively. Those who have problems managing their weight tend to lack assertiveness and avoid interpersonal conflict. Refusing other people's requests or needs is difficult, and getting or giving criticism is often the instigator of overeating.

To keep weight off permanently requires being able to cope effectively with stress. Stress increases when your relationships aren't working. Relationships that work are a source of satisfaction and nurturance. When your relationships are happy, your need to use food to deal with stress is reduced. Successful weight management is more likely when you are able to communicate effectively and manage the inevitable conflicts that occur between people.

References

1.   McKay, M., David, M. & Fanning, P. (1983). *Messages: The Communication Book*. Oakland, CA: New Harbinger Publications.

2.   Gravitz, H.L., & Bowden, J.D. (1985). *Guide to Recovery: A Book for Adult Children of Alcoholics*. Holmes Beach, FL: Learning Publications.

3.   Zimbardo, P.G. (1977). *Shyness*. Reading, MA: Addison-Wesley.

Chapter 7

Overcoming Depression and Anxiety

EMOTIONS ARE FEELINGS with labels such as love, hate, joy, distress, fear, anger, shame, and so forth. The person who is experiencing emotion tends to feel stirred up or excited. When the emotion is sadness or depression, the person may feel slowed down or unable to move. It is generally easy to tell what emotion a person is feeling, just by looking at her face and watching how she acts.

In addition to being a feeling state that is associated with some kind of observable behavior, emotion involves cognition—thinking. To be able to feel emotional about something, you must first perceive that something and understand it. Thus, if someone says something insulting about you, you must hear about the insult and decide it is something to get upset about, before you will actually feel upset. It may seem that something that happens causes you to feel a certain way, but actually how you feel is the result of how you think—the meaning you give to events.

There are times when remembering something can bring back old feelings. Memories, in the form of images or symbols, can have an emotional charge. How feelings become associated or bonded with images in memory is not understood. Often memories that are painful are not readily available to consciousness, but can be pulled back into consciousness by certain events.

When an event triggers some emotion, you can take control over your emotional reaction in a variety of ways. You can interpret the event so that you do not automatically get upset. Or if you do get upset initially, you can use self-talk to calm yourself down. You can even change your mind about what something from the past means, and thus alter how it once affected you. By changing your thinking, you can alter how you feel.

Emotions also produce a physical reaction in the body—tension, arousal, or in some cases sluggishness. You can gain control of the physical arousal of emotion by using such techniques as deep breathing, progressive relaxation, meditation, exercise, or guided imagery.

130

You can also take steps to make it less likely that upsetting events will happen. By staying away from people and places that have caused trouble in the past, you reduce the likelihood of such problems in the future.

Emotions triggered by painful memories, especially if they are of traumatic events, can present some special difficulties. These may intrude themselves on your awareness—even if you don't want to recall them, they may enter consciousness. This may happen through distressing dreams or flashbacks—the experience of being back in the event at the present moment.

Often such memories are accompanied by difficulty sleeping or concentrating. Likewise, one may startle at the least thing—a loud noise or sudden change. If such memories become too disruptive to your life and you aren't able to cope with them yourself, the help of a professional therapist should be sought.

In most cases, there is much you can do to gain control of your emotions. You can refuse to dwell on upsetting thoughts, or you can take a different point of view about events. When a difficult memory comes to mind, you can try turning your thoughts elsewhere. Later in this chapter you will learn how to use imagery to cope with emotions and painful memories.

Emotions, whether they come from your perception of events or from memories, can make weight management more difficult. Particularly problematic are the painful emotions of depression, anxiety, anger, and loneliness. Emotions can lead to inappropriate eating, particularly snacking on high-calorie foods. While not every weight problem is caused by emotional eating, understanding and learning to cope more effectively with difficult emotions can make life generally more satisfying, and is likely to increase your chances for successful weight management in the long term.

Depression

Many people with weight problems suffer from various degrees of depression. As a result, they experience feelings of helplessness, hopelessness, and personal inadequacy. Depression can range from relatively mild to quite severe, with serious implications for mental health. If depression gets bad enough, the sufferer may even wish she were dead.

Depression is often triggered by real or imagined misfortunes, failures, defeats, or losses. Feeling unhappy or depressed in response to such events is normal and "healthy," and does not usually indicate poor mental health. Such depression usually improves with time. However, over-reacting, or not reacting at all to misfortune, or being unable to control the expression of emotion in response to events, can be a sign of deeper problems.

Sometimes depression doesn't seem to have a clear, external cause. There appears to be no triggering event, no real loss or defeat. The depressed person may say, "I feel miserable, but I have no reason to feel unhappy. I really have nothing to complain about, so why do I feel depressed?"

Symptoms of depression include crying a lot, feeling depressed most of the time, having problems sleeping, overeating or having little appetite, having little interest in activities that used to give pleasure, and experiencing fatigue or agitation. Sometimes depression is experienced as physical symptoms—headaches, backaches, gastrointestinal disturbance, etc.

The depressed person usually shows a lack of self-confidence, engages in self-blame, feels isolated and forsaken, has a pessimistic outlook on life, and dwells on past events. He or she often experiences feelings of inferiority and guilt as well as partial or total helplessness.

When these symptoms appear, the depressed person is likely to be helped by getting emotional support from others (including a therapist) and learning to change her thinking so that she can help herself out of the depression hole she is in.

Depression that is persistent—lasting weeks or months—or recurring, is likely to be unhealthy. There are a number of important signs that depression is severe and needs the help of a mental health professional: waking two hours or more before your usual time of arising, having a feeling of dread at having to face the day, losing more than ten pounds without trying, or feeling either agitated or unable to move. Even if you experience only one or two of these, you should seek help.

Possible Causes of Unhealthy Depression

Unhealthy depression can result from a number of things. In rare cases, there can be an organic cause, but most of the time, depression comes from the kinds of interactions you have or have had with others.

Some kinds of depression have their roots in the past—perhaps a parent or caregiver failed you repeatedly in some important way. Depression can be the result of being in a bad situation—one in which you are emotionally, physically, or sexually abused. Depression is also triggered by losses or the failure to attain adequate satisfaction in life.

Some people who have had a low-level of depression for many years even come to think that feeling the way they do is "normal." For them, depression has become an integral part of their self-concept. As the result of feeling "down" for years, the possibility they might feel better no longer seems an option for them.

In virtually all kinds of depression, the way in which you think—your beliefs and self-talk—contribute to depression. When you are depressed, it is hard to remember the good things in life. Thoughts almost automatically become pessimistic. To beat depression, you need to overcome the tendency toward negativity and actively promote positive thinking.

Physiological or Organic Causes

In some cases, unhealthy depression is the result of physiological or organic causes—a brain tumor, a stroke, dysfunction in the brain, chemical imbalance in the body, and so forth. Sometimes it is quite difficult to get a physician to order appropriate tests for assessing a possible biological basis for depression because of a tendency to assume, in the absence of obvious physical abnormalities, that depression is primarily psychological. Usually this is true, but for some people depression does have a physiological cause.

If you suffer depression that is severe and chronic, has no apparent cause or is increasing in severity, and especially if you also are experiencing disorientation or lapses in memory, insist on having appropriate tests done to rule out a possible physiological cause for the depression. A psychiatrist or neurologist can order such tests. Psychologists and mental health professionals without an M.D. cannot do so directly, although they may be able to arrange for such tests.

Once a physiological or organic cause of severe depression has been ruled out, you may confidently pursue psychological treatment. A competent mental health professional will work with you to rule out physiological and organic causes before or together with any psychological intervention. Once a physiological cause is ruled out, a combination of antidepressant medication, together with psychotherapy, may be appropriate.

The Early Parent/Child Relationship

For some people who have had a long-standing weight problem, depression may have its roots in the early parent/child interactions, including the feeding relationship, the level of protectiveness exhibited by the parents, or the degree of love and acceptance conveyed to the child.

The feeding relationship that exists between the mother and infant is a crucial early influence on emotional development.[1,2] It is in this mother/child interaction that the child gains awareness of what she is feeling, learns that she can get what she wants and needs, and develops trust that someone will provide for her. The child has survival needs—oxygen, food, water, rest—and the need for acceptance and love. The infant and child depend totally on the parents to satisfy these needs.

In a positive feeding relationship, the mother consistently attends to the child's rhythms and signals of hunger and satiety so that the timing of feeding, amount of food given, preferences, and pacing are appropriate for that particular child. The mother takes care to calm the child and respond to her emotional needs as well.

When the mother and child are consistently successful in this way, the feeding relationship contributes to the development of appropriate feelings of love, acceptance, and security that are vital to emotional health. If this feeding relationship is not dependably positive, however, the child, and later the adult, may suffer emotional disturbance, including depression.

One way the feeding relationship can be detrimental to the child is if the feeding mother resents the child, or thinks how great her life could be without the baby. The child senses this. An infant is endowed with the ability to perceive nonverbal signals and feel whether or not she is loved by the feeding mother or maternal substitute. Indeed, it has been shown that infants who are merely fed but not provided with love and touching fail to thrive.

Feeding provides not only food, but also love, security, and pleasure. When the feeding mother is inconsistent or rejecting, the child becomes anxiety-ridden and fears mother will abandon her. As a result, the child may confuse contractions of the stomach related to food deprivation with those related to emotional states. Later in life, she may react by craving food whenever she is depressed or worried.

Likewise, if the mother is domineering or insensitive to the child's needs, the feeding relationship can be detrimental. Normally, the amount of food an infant will take corresponds, more or less, to the infant's physiological needs. A domineering mother, on the other hand, or one that slavishly follows the advice of well-meaning others without paying attention to her child's nonverbal cues, may force the child to eat past the point of satiety. Or an impatient or insensitive mother may terminate feeding before the child is fully satisfied.

When the child's needs are not accurately identified and gratified, or these needs conflict with what her mother wants to give her, the child may become confused about her physical sensations and anxious about having her needs met.

Some parents reward the infant and child for eating without hunger. The infant learns to eat for mother's smile, and the young child learns to eat in order to please her parents. Some children come to believe that the more they eat, the more their parents will love them. Eventually they become conditioned to eating large quantities of food even when they are not hungry. Later attempts to curb this behavior may produce fear of maternal disapproval and guilt feelings for disobeying mother.

One result of a detrimental feeding relationship can be that the child becomes an adult who has not learned to tell the difference between emotional cues and hunger. Indeed, it has been shown that overweight people react more to emotional events and are more likely to engage in emotional eating, particularly snacking, than are normal weight people.

It may be that some obese people do not learn the difference between true hunger and emotional arousal. Indeed, studies have demonstrated that some obese people cannot distinguish between physiological hunger signaled by stomach contractions and cravings for food not related to hunger.

Parents who are overly protective also set the stage for emotional difficulty and possibly eating problems later in life. The parents' own insecurity and emotional shortcomings may get translated into over-protectiveness that can extend to feeding as well. The child who is not allowed to explore, take the initiative, and fend for herself will find it more difficult to develop the self-confidence necessary to become a fully functioning adult.

When a parent consistently inhibits the child's exploration, the child does not learn to experience, interpret, and trust her own reality. The covert message given to the child by an overprotective parent is, "You can't do it yourself. You are too clumsy, stupid, or inadequate." If this control is extended to eating behavior, the child does not learn to know or respect her own signals of food regulation, and learns instead to regulate feeding on the basis of the interaction with her parents. Such over-protectiveness causes the child to develop low self-esteem, and to feel unable to influence how things turn out.

To make matters worse, the overprotective parent is often very critical of the child as well. If the child becomes overweight, either as a result of trying to please the parent or because of not learning to manage her own eating behavior, the parent may alternate his or her overprotective posture with bursts of hostility and criticism.

If the child reaches adolescence and is overweight, peers are likely to join in the criticism, further discouraging self-esteem. The child may be torn between the already-established desire to overeat to please her mother of yesterday, and the desire to avoid the criticism of peers and her mother of today.

Lack of love and acceptance of the child on the part of a parent can lead to emotional as well as eating difficulties. Because of this, some obese people may actually feel "starved for love," and use eating in an attempt to fill the void. Seeking an elusive sense of being loved and accepted by others, they may alternately reach out to and then reject other people. Although they desperately want love and acceptance, they don't really believe they deserve love. They may adopt the Groucho Marx attitude that "I wouldn't join any club that would have me as a member," and decide that anyone who could love them must be wrong, stupid, or worthless.

Some people who are overweight withdraw from social relations. If they have invested a lot of emotional energy trying to gain acceptance and love, and still have not been able to satisfy these needs, they may feel close to emotional bankruptcy. As a result, they withdraw, claiming that they wish to avoid criticism, derogatory comments, and rejection. Having isolated themselves, their depression and feelings of helplessness and hopelessness deepen.

When such a situation exists, overeating can fuel self-hate: "I'm so unlovable I may as well make myself fat and repulsive!" Anger at the world for not responding to needs for acceptance and love, and anger at oneself for being weak and helpless are directed inward. Overeating becomes self-punishment and obesity one's "just reward."

Bad Situations

Depression can also be fostered by a bad situation—one in which a person is physically, emotionally, or sexually abused by someone or by the "system." As a result, self-esteem is eroded, and the person feels rejected or helpless.

The perpetrator may be a parent, spouse, child, boss, co-worker, neighbor, or bureaucrat. Examples of bad situations include: being married to or living with a spouse-beater, an alcoholic, a drug abuser, or a person who engages in continuous criticism, blaming, or verbal abuse; working for a person or organization that makes excessive demands without adequate physical or psychological relief; being economically deprived or dependent; or being socially repressed or discriminated against. When a person is caught in a bad situation and does not perceive a way out, depression is a likely result.

In an attempt to cope with her misery, the victim of a bad situation may turn to alcohol to give her the illusion of power over the situation. Intoxication dulls the pain, and she may believe herself to be more attractive, sociable, ready to embrace the entire world, and able to bring about an easy solution to all ills. Alternatively, she may turn to prescription or street drugs. Or she may turn to food, using it in a similar way to push away the pain and the feelings of being unloved, unaccepted, unacknowledged, weak, and helpless.

Unfortunately, such misuse of alcohol, drugs, or food only makes things worse, and further enmeshes her in her problem. While such self-destructive behaviors may provide a short-term escape, ultimately they only deepen depression, and force her to seek ever-increasing measures for relief.

Failure to Attain Satisfaction

Sometimes having a weight problem is a way of avoiding having to deal with life problems. Losing weight may sound like a good idea, but having a weight problem can have its rewards. Worrying about weight provides a distraction from such problems as being in a non-supportive relationship or a dead-end job, as well as a good excuse for inaction, passivity, and failure.

Successful weight management would force having to deal head-on with the real issues. Continued failure at managing weight becomes a self-fulfilling prophesy. Depression, then, finds its roots not only in the failure to manage weight, but also in the failure to attain deeper satisfaction or contentment in life.

Chronic, Low-Level Depression

In some cases, depression can actually become part of the self-concept, especially if it has existed at a low level for several years. Generally, this "down" mood begins in childhood, adolescence, or early adult life. Such depression no longer has an identifiable cause. Rather the person suffering from it never expects much joy from life. Feeling depressed or irritable most of the day, more days than not, seems "normal" to such people.

An example of this kind of "depressive personality" is Maggie, whose parents sent her to a prestigious, live-in weight reduction program in the hope that losing weight would help relieve the depression that had plagued her for years. Maggie came back thinner, but still depressed. Eventually, Maggie regained the weight she had lost. Being thinner had not made her life more rewarding, and it seemed pointless to keep up the effort required to maintain goal weight.

Depression and the "Impostor" Phenomenon

Sometimes depression is suffered by very successful people who have difficulty coming to terms with their own success. They understand that they have achieved the trappings of success and are generally well-respected by their peers, but they don't feel loved and accepted for who they really are.

Sometimes such people attribute their success to sources outside themselves—luck, timing, good looks, hard work, social connections—rather than to their own skill or intelligence. They negate any evidence that contradicts this perception, believing that they are, in fact, a fraud and a fake.

Those most vulnerable to this problem tend to believe that others don't truly know them for who they are. In some cases, they achieve in areas that are not typical for their families. As a result, they may feel that somehow they have disappointed the family.

Perhaps they have tried all their life to please one or both parents, but have never felt the parent's approval. Even though outsiders acknowledge their success, the person feels empty. Whatever the source, the "impostor" is beset with depression, anxiety, and frustration, from alternately fearing exposure of their "fraudulent" status, and working furiously to cover it up.

Beliefs and Thinking

The beliefs people hold and the way they think contribute to depression. Aaron Beck, a psychiatrist known for his work on depression, views it as the result of three types of beliefs or thought patterns.[3] The first is a negative view of self, by which he means that the depressed person sees herself as inadequate, unlovable, or unworthy. When something unpleasant happens, she blames herself for having some physical, mental, or moral defect. As a result, she underestimates herself, believing that she does not have what it takes to attain real happiness or at least contentment.

Secondly, the depressed person sees the world as presenting unsurmountable obstacles. Her thinking is characterized by distorted reasoning and "thinking traps." She finds evidence for her unworthiness and confirmation of her faults by filtering out any "good news" about herself and focusing only on her failures. She tends to take things personally and interpret even neutral remarks as criticism. By establishing unrealistic standards for herself, she frequently feels overwhelmed. Because she tends to discount those successes she does have, she suffers persistently low self-esteem.

Finally, the depressed person is likely to view the future in a negative way. She anticipates that current suffering will continue indefinitely. She expects failure. The future looks as bleak as her current reality.

Assessing Your Depression

The following self-test, *Are You Depressed?,* will help you determine the degree to which you may be suffering from depression, and whether you should seek professional help. Use your scores on this self-test, together with the symptoms given earlier indicating severe depression, to determine whether you should seek professional help for depression.

The self-test refers to 18 areas of experience in your life, followed by a series of descriptions that shade from "normal" to increasingly indicative of depression. Rate each of the items by choosing the number that is closest to the description that best represents your experience over the last several weeks.

For the description "same as usual," refer to how you were feeling the last time you felt happy and not depressed, or to what you think is normal for most people. Circle one number only for each item, and do not skip any items.

Overcoming Depression

The first step in coping with depression is to realize that sometimes sadness is a normal and appropriate reaction to events, and that it is likely to pass in time. Keep reminding yourself that this will pass and that you will adjust.

When depression does not pass in a reasonable amount of time, when it is severe, or when the reaction to a stressful event is not appropriate—you overreact or under-react to an event—you may need the assistance of a competent mental health professional.

If the situation you are in is contributing to your feeling depressed, you may need the help of agencies and organizations set up for this purpose. A call to your local community mental health agency or a look in your telephone book can result in your getting in touch with an appropriate group for your needs.

For example, Al-Anon provides support to families of alcoholics, even if the alcoholic is not himself in treatment. There are also groups or organizations that provide support and advice for battered women, for those who feel suicidal, for parents who get upset with their children, and a variety

Self-Test 7.1

Are You Depressed?

1. Sleep pattern:

0	1	2	3	4
Same as usual		Fitful		Wake early, can't sleep; (or sleep a lot more than usual)

2. Energy level:

0	1	2	3	4
Normal ebb and flow		Tired a lot		No energy at all, (or alternating very high energy and no energy)

3. Eating and appetite:

0	1	2	3	4
Same as usual		Decreased (or increased)		No appetite at all (or overeating a lot)

4. Weight over the past month:

0	1	2	3	4
Steady		Lost a little (or gained a litttle) without trying		Lost a lot (or gained a lot) without trying

5. Desire for sex:

0	1	2	3	4
Same as usual		Decreased		Not at all interested

6. Ability to work:

0	1	2	3	4
Same as usual		Difficult to get motivated or concentrate		Unable to function

7. Interest in other activities or people:

0	1	2	3	4
Same as usual		Less than usual		No interest at all

8. Evaluation of personal accomplishments:

0	1	2	3	4
Same as usual		Dissatisfied		Feel like a total failure

9. Evaluation of self:

0	1	2	3	4
Acceptable		Dissatisfied with self		Hate myself

10. Perspective on future:

0	1	2	3	4
Things will work out		Discouraged		Completely hopeless

(continued)

Self-Test 7.1

Are You Depressed? (continued)

11. Experience of life:

0	1	2	3	4
Satisfied		Somewhat disappointed		Totally dissatisfied

12. Reaction to actual misfortune:

0	1	2	3	4
Mildly upset		Very upset		Extremely upset (or feel nothing)

13. Feelings of "sadness":

0	1	2	3	4
Rarely sad		Sometimes sad		Sad or unhappy all or most or the time

14. Sensitivity to irritation:

0	1	2	3	4
Same as usual		More irritable than usual		Very irritable and easily upset

15. Duration of depressed feelings:

0	1	2	3	4
Lifts in a few days or weeks		Some days it seems better, but depression never really goes away		Seems like I've always been depressed

16. Apparent reason for negative feelings when I have them:

0	1	2	3	4
A specific event or crisis		A difficult situation that keeps persisting		Don't know

of other such problems. Or check *Appendix A* of this book and call the self-help clearinghouse nearest you to determine local resources that might be of help.

With or without professional help, there is much you can do to help yourself.

1.   *Change your thinking.* When you are depressed, you have difficulty focusing on anything but the negative. All you can think of is how bad things are, how bad they've been, and how bad they are going to continue to be. You tend to label everything that happens or that has happened as awful and hopeless. Your "thinking traps" color everything. In particular, feeling depressed is maintained by the following tendencies:

• The tendency to label things negatively, rather than challenging your first assumption and trying to find a more positive way of interpreting something that happens.

Self-Test 7.1

Are You Depressed? (continued)

17. Crying:

         0   1   2   3   4

Same as usual   Cry a lot   Want to cry but can't anymore; numb

18. Thoughts of killing myself:

         0   1   2   3   4

Never have such thoughts   Thought of it but wouldn't really do it   Seriously thought about it

Totals: _____ + _____ + _____ + _____ + _____ = _____

Score Interpretation

Total Score	Levels of Depression
0–10	Normal ups and downs.
11–20	Mild mood disturbance; if it persists, it would be helpful to seek professional assistance.
21–35	Moderate depression; professional assistance is recommended
Over 35	Severe depression; professional assistance is strongly advised.

- The tendency to draw a conclusion when there is little or no evidence to support it (e.g., "I never do anything right"), or to draw a conclusion based on only one incident (e.g., "I got out of breath after only five minutes on my exercise bike; I don't think I can exercise"), rather than evaluating all of the evidence more objectively.

- The tendency to take details out of context, ignoring other aspects of the situation, and then conceptualizing the whole experience on the basis of the one detail (e.g., "I ate a cookie when I shouldn't have; my whole week is shot"), rather than adopting a more balanced point of view that includes the "good news" as well as the "bad news."

- The tendency to relate external events to yourself when there is no basis for making such a connection (e.g., "When she said she couldn't understand how some people could let themselves go like that, she was really talking about me"), rather than interpreting the event as a statement about the other person.

You need to become aware of such tendencies, and whenever you find yourself thinking this way, change what you are saying to yourself. Review the information in Chapter 4, *Using Self-Talk Effectively,* about changing self-talk and using self-instructional statements, as well as the information in Chapter 3 on thinking traps.

In particular, it is important to develop self-acceptance. Even when you make mistakes (and everyone does), this can be seen as information to help you change so you can ultimately get what you want. Blaming or judging yourself harshly as bad or morally deficient doesn't help. Being accountable, by assessing what you did or didn't do that contributed to the way things turned out, does help.

When you can accept yourself, despite your faults and the mistakes you have made, you feel better. When you get down on yourself, you make yourself feel down and depressed. To become more self-accepting, you have to become somewhat detached from things. You need to take life, and yourself, a little less seriously. When you "ease up" on yourself, life tends to go better, and your experience of life improves.

2.   *Get active.* The more depressed one feels, the more one withdraws from the world and from the activities that used to give pleasure. It is as if the depressed person were trying to escape from reality or reduce the level of stimulation she feels.

Paradoxically, an important step in letting go of depression is to accept the fact that you are depressed and get out and get more involved anyway. Create opportunities for purposeful activity in your life by scheduling your day. Plan one day at a time. Do one task at a time. Don't worry about being perfect; just get involved in doing.

Choose activities that absorb your interest and help your concentration—such as cooking, cleaning, taking walks, filing, making phone calls, writing letters, etc. If a task seems too overwhelming, go to a more simple task. Be flexible. Be kind to yourself.

3.   *Exercise.* Research has shown that exercise is at least as effective as prescription drugs in helping to lift depression, and increasingly exercise is being prescribed as a means of coping with depression. Regular, vigorous exercise causes the brain to produce endorphins—natural tranquilizers that help to normalize moods.

It isn't necessary to become a "jock." Just getting out for a walk is a good place to start. You might consider joining a fitness class or a dance class. It helps to plan to do exercise with a partner or to join a class, because the other people involved provide motivation for you to continue.

4. *Change your environment.* Sometimes the situation you are in is an important contributor to your depression. For example, having to constantly reprimand or limit a young child's behavior can drain your emotional resources. It may be necessary to take steps to change your environment.

In the case of the overactive child, it could mean "child-proofing" the home by putting some things under lock and key. As another example, if there are arguments over which TV program to watch, getting another TV could help. In the most drastic case, it may mean your getting away, at least temporarily, from the source of irritation. If you need to move out, you may have to contact an appropriate agency or organization that specializes in providing such assistance.

Taking such actions is especially hard to do when you are depressed, because it is difficult to believe that anything you do can make a difference in how you feel. You may have difficulty thinking of options for action, or you may feel so heavy or burdened that taking any action seems impossible. Depression often immobilizes your ability to act at all.

To get moving, you must talk differently to yourself. Tell yourself that you *can* take action to help yourself. Reject thoughts that are self-critical, that see problems as insurmountable, or that expect things to turn out badly.

Talk to others whom you respect, and ask for their suggestions and support. Just taking these small steps will begin to prove to you that you can act effectively, and this will help to alter your conviction that there is no solution. Remind yourself that even small steps are evidence of progress, and focus on continuing to cope one day at a time.

5. *Experience and let go.* This is especially important when the source of depression is rooted in the early parent/child relationship. Some people were victimized as children by verbal, physical, or sexual abuse. Others may have failed to get the love or approval they always wanted from a parent. Even the best parents are deficient from time to time with their children.

The hurts from parental failures or childhood difficulties can become the hidden cause of problems with others in present-day interactions for the now-adult children. Old anger because "Dad never told me he loved me. . ." or "Mom was always too busy with her things. . ." may be expressed in many ways in current relationships.

The emotions associated with these hurts and injuries are valid and need to be experienced fully. When the feelings have been experienced and validated—that is, accepted as legitimate—then the process of letting go can begin. To let go of old hurts so that they no longer cripple one's life requires accepting and grieving the losses of the past, and gradually becoming more able to reinvest energy into the present and the future.

In an effort to clean up the relationship, or to try and change their parents, some people try confronting a parent with the sources of old hurts, seeking an explanation or some validation of self. Unfortunately, this rarely works. The parent has his or her own views on the matter, which usually differ from yours, and may react with hurt or anger at the implication he or she was not a "good parent."

You can, however, undertake such a confrontation and seek a resolution by using imagery in a particular way. In the next section, *6. Use Imagery to Elevate Your Mood,* you are given detailed instructions for doing self-guided imagery.

Choose a time when you will not be interrupted for 30 to 60 minutes, and then settle yourself comfortably in a chair or on a bed. Allow yourself to relax deeply. Then bring into your imagination a scene in which you confront your parent with your concerns. Imagine yourself saying what you have to say, but be sure to listen to what your parent has to say to you in your imagination.

If you feel angry or hurt, or some other emotion during the imagery process, allow yourself to experience these feelings fully and then to let go of them. Experiencing fully the emotions connected to old memories is important. This is part of the grieving process that will allow you to let go of the hurts. Another exercise for letting go of past hurts involves using two chairs, one for you and one empty one in which you imagine your parent sitting. Place the chairs fairly close together facing each other. Sitting in one chair and imagining one of your parents in the other, say whatever it is you have to say to your parent. Then change chairs and respond as if you were your parent, sitting in the other chair. Again, be emotionally honest, and be willing to forgive and let go.

You may have to repeat the imagery or chairs exercise a number of times before you feel you have processed the emotions adequately. It helps to have a therapist or counselor with whom you can talk and continue to work through your feelings.

In anticipating doing either the imagery exercise or the empty chair exercise, you may be concerned that your emotions will overwhelm you. This is especially true for anger. Anger is an upsetting emotion that may be associated with abuse you have suffered. It is also frightening. You may fear that if you let yourself experience it, you'll lose control and actually hurt someone. That's why people tend to repress anger.

The problem is, repressing anger contributes to depression. And what's more, repressed anger is unpredictable—it can explode at any time. When it does, it is often uncontrollable. Alternatively, giving yourself permission to be angry without making any judgments about your feelings will help diffuse and dissipate the build-up of pent-up rage.

6. *Use imagery to elevate your mood.* Imagery is a technique you can use to elevate your mood and to cope with depression. (Later you will learn how imagery can also be used to gain a better understanding of perplexing situations, to restructure your thinking, to build personal confidence, to resolve a difficult situation, and to mentally rehearse new behavior patterns.)

Using imagery simply means being able to "see" pictures in your mind. Some people can imagine very vividly, while others sense images more than "see" them. Everyone has the ability to call up mental images, even though they may think they don't. Imagination is so much a part of human experience that you may be unaware that you do it all the time. The pictures you see in your mind's eye when you are trying to give someone directions are one example of your ability to do imagery.

The basic instructions for doing imagery are as follows:

1.   *Get relaxed.* Find a private place, one where you will not be interrupted for a period of time—usually at least 15 to 20 minutes. It helps to get settled comfortably in a chair or on a bed. Close your eyes and relax. (See the section beginning on page 152 of this chapter that discusses how to elicit the relaxation response.) Then use your imagination.

Remember, there is no right or wrong way to do imagery. Some people readily see pictures in their minds, whereas others tend more to sense them. The more you do imagery, the better able you will be to create vivid pictures in your mind.

2.   *Mentally picture a relaxing scene.* The relaxing scene you bring to mind for this purpose should promote calmness, tranquility, or enjoyment for you. Examples might include skiing on a beautiful slope, hiking on a secluded trail, sailing on a sunny lake, walking on a secluded beach, or lying in the green grass of a quiet meadow. The image should include as much sensory detail as possible—sounds, colors, temperature, smell, touch, and motion. The more enjoyable the sensations and the greater the intensity of the pleasure, the easier it will be for you to relax and achieve a peaceful, happy feeling.

You may find it easier to do imagery if you carefully write out the details of the scene you want to imagine. Then record it on an audiocassette tape to play back while you are relaxing. (When you are recording your scene on tape, be careful to speak slowly and in a relaxing tone of voice.)

3.   *Allow yourself to become involved in the scene.* Give yourself permission to enjoy this purposeful daydreaming. Continue until you have enjoyed this mental imaging sufficiently and are feeling relaxed and satisfied. Then open your eyes, stretch your muscles, and continue your day with an improved perspective.

4.   *Practice doing imagery.* Do this at least once a day, repeating steps 1 and 2 each time, until you feel confident in your ability to improve your mood by using imagery. If you wish, try different kinds of images to alter your mood.

Stimulating imagery can make you feel more energetic. To overcome the inertia that often accompanies depression, use imagery to "see" yourself jumping up and down on a trampoline, going higher and higher as you experience the feeling of flying. Or imagine yourself playing a superb game of tennis. Mentally experience yourself reaching smoothly for every shot and getting it, no matter how difficult. Let yourself feel the exhilaration of playing well.

You can do a great deal to overcome depression on your own. Understanding what depression is and how it can be created is a helpful beginning in learning how to cope with it.

Changing the way you think is particularly important for coping better with depression. Getting active and doing things also helps. Sometimes this means changing your environment. Another way to get active is to exercise. Also, allowing yourself to experience and work through emotions, especially anger, that are related to childhood experiences can be very important. Finally, using self-guided imagery to elevate moods may be helpful.

In some cases, depression needs the attention of a trained professional—a psychiatrist, psychologist, or other licensed mental health professional. Reaching out for professional help should never be a source of embarrassment or shame; it is a sign of strength.

Anxiety

June had succeeded in losing 65 pounds and had maintained her goal weight for six months. One of the ways she used to maintain her success was to be a lecturer, teaching others how to lose weight with a well-known weight control program. Even so, June battled anxiety.

"Every day I wake up and I'm afraid to get out of bed. I'm afraid this will be the day it will begin. This will be the day I'll start regaining weight. I worry about what I'll eat that day, and I'm afraid to eat anything. I'm afraid to get on the scale, and if I've gained a pound I almost get hysterical. If I regain the weight it will be awful and horrible, but I can't stand this much longer. I think it may be better to regain the weight and get it over with, than live my life this way."

Joanne, an older student pursuing a masters degree, was unable to start weight reduction efforts because of her anxiety. She explained that she had gone on diets before, and she just couldn't face the inevitable hunger pangs that trying to lose weight would bring. Even the anticipation of having to diet made her hands shake and caused a tension headache.

As a struggling graduate student, she couldn't afford to have her ability to concentrate impaired, and that's just what being hungry did. So Joanne kept putting off doing anything about her weight; but then when she looked in the mirror, she got upset and anxious because she felt she had to do something about her weight soon.

Gayle was a former beauty queen who had been a contestant in the Miss America contest and subsequently gained 125 pounds. She was overwhelmed with depression because of her weight, but paralyzed by anxiety at the thought of undertaking weight reduction.

She explained through her tears that she couldn't stand how people had treated her when she was a beauty queen. They seemed to relate to her appearance, rather than to who she really was, and she often felt like just a sex object. Thinking about losing weight and having to deal with such treatment and the expectations that other people put on her made her stomach tighten and her hands turn cold and clammy. Yet the prospect of staying fat was equally awful.

Just trying to get around made her short of breath, and she tired easily. Even though the few friends she had were very sympathetic, Gayle didn't socialize much, and she was preoccupied with her problem. There seemed to be no satisfactory solution; losing weight or not losing weight were equally bad alternatives. She suffered repeated spells of crying. She felt helpless and powerless to do anything about her problem.

Paula gained 100 pounds shortly after her second marriage. Periodically she would attempt weight reduction, but very shortly would develop severe attacks of anxiety, and give up. "I don't know what happens. I have nothing to be afraid of, but I start losing a little weight, and this huge fear that I can't identify grips me. My hands start to shake, the muscles in the back of my neck get tight, and I feel as if I can't breathe. Nothing seems to help. I can't concentrate, and finally I just quit trying to lose weight. Only then does the fear go away."

The Experience of Anxiety

In contrast to depression, which is typically a response to loss, anxiety is a fear response to threat. The threat may be real, something that is likely to happen or is actually impending. June was concerned with the real threat of regaining weight.

Anxiety can also be the result both of perceiving a threat where none exists, or of exaggerating the importance of a real threat. Joanne's anxiety was produced by her concern that trying to lose weight would mean having to endure hunger.

Anxiety can result from a traumatic event that produces painful memories, and continuing to relive these in one's imagination. Gayle was paralyzed about weight reduction because of her painful memories of being slim, but at the same time she felt threatened by the very real health problems she was experiencing from being severely overweight.

Or threat can be something that is not identifiable. Paula could not identify a real threat. In her case, the source of threat was blocked from her awareness. The source of unidentifiable threat may be repressed traumatic memories or unconscious fears.

Typically, anxiety is experienced as some kind of physical arousal—nervousness, tenseness, or agitation. Symptoms of anxiety that can be debilitating include sweating, nausea, shortness of breath, chest pain, chills or flushes, dizziness or unsteady feelings, or trembling and shaking. There may be difficulty concentrating. As these symptoms become more intense, the anxiety may actually escalate into a panic attack.

The severely anxious person may become a hypochondriac, develop phobias, and experience depression as well as anxiety. The cause of severe anxiety is a combination of biochemical disorder, psychological complications, and environmental stress. Proper treatment involves a thorough medical evaluation and medical treatment, combined in most cases with psychological treatment.

In all cases of anxiety, the way one thinks contributes to the experience of anxiety. Worries about what might happen characterize anxious thinking. Fear of being criticized, fear of others' evaluation of you, fear of not being able to perform, fear of the unexpected—are just some of the worries that bedevil the anxious person. Over and over again, she asks herself, "What if. . .?" Because she needs to control what she can't control, she feels increasingly out of control—and more anxious.

When Anxiety Becomes Disruptive

Some anxiety is normal and appropriate when it is a response to a real threat. In fact, a low level of anxiety can actually improve certain types of performance. For example, experiencing anxiety because of a forthcoming job evaluation interview is normal, and can help prompt the employee to prepare herself mentally and emotionally for the experience.

On the other hand, anxiety is not normal if it inhibits the ability to function, or if it disrupts effective action. By dwelling on the potential threat of regaining weight, and repeatedly thinking catastrophizing thoughts, June exaggerated the threat in her mind, thereby escalating her anxiety levels to so high a level that she experienced fear and dread each day. Her ability to function day to day was being compromised, and the only solution she could see was to give up and regain the weight in order to relieve the emotional tension.

Joanne's anxiety kept her from undertaking a serious weight reduction effort, and she kept looking for a quick solution that would avoid hunger. As a result, she fell prey to a variety of weight reduction swindles, including body wraps, starch blockers, and appetite reducing pills. Lacking success in losing weight, she withdrew further from her friends and social network.

In most cases, the memory of a traumatic event is relived in memory a little bit at a time, so that eventually the experience is absorbed in a healthy way. Sometimes, however, the emotions connected with a traumatic event are so strong, and the memory of the event brings back the emotion so vividly that it is not absorbed in a healthy way. As a result, the person attempts to avoid re-exposure to the painful situation. Gayle was reportedly so traumatized by her experience as a beauty queen that she reacted defensively, ensuring that she could not be treated like a beauty queen again—as a result she became severely obese.

What is not known is whether Gayle's reaction to being treated as a "sexual object" as a beauty queen might be connected to a deeper, more traumatic event in her childhood, which is not yet consciously available to her. Sometimes the mind defends itself by denying a traumatic or painful experience and blocking it out of awareness. Eventually the experience either may resurface on its own, perhaps in dreams, or be brought to consciousness by another event.

When Paula participated in an imagery process, the traumatic circumstances of her first husband's death came back to her, and she realized that she had never allowed herself to really grieve. Her response to severe loss had been to avoid all reminders of loss. Because she had not "worked through" the loss, the threat still existed, but it was blocked from consciousness. For her, eating was a way to push out of consciousness anxious feelings for which she had no explanation; the memory was blocked from her awareness because it was too painful.

Adaptive Anxiety

When anxiety is kept within reasonable limits, it serves as an early warning system that allows you to adjust and adapt. Anxiety allows you to prepare in advance for dealing with a real threat by giving you the opportunity to deal with it in small doses.

Going back to the earlier example, you are likely to feel anxious about an impending job evaluation interview. For some time prior to the interview, you typically ignore it, until it is almost upon you. That is, you defend yourself against the threat by not admitting it to consciousness until the last possible minute.

When you do finally let yourself think about it, you may imagine the worst possible outcome—that you get fired. After rehashing this outcome in your mind several times over, you may begin to focus on more realistic outcomes—that your boss offers some compliments for your work and some suggestions on how to improve.

In essence, you may prepare for an anxiety-producing event by first thinking about the worst possible outcome, and then gradually imagining less and less stressful outcomes. When you are able to deal with a threat in small doses, your ability to cope with it is increased. The anxiety you experience in this way is normal and appropriate.

Similarly, it is normal and adaptive to experience anxiety with regard to an earlier stressful event that you had not anticipated, and with which you were suddenly confronted. Recalling such a stressful experience, and reexperiencing some of that anxiety now is part of the natural process of integrating the experience and resolving the associated emotion.

The subconscious approach to mastering the stress associated with a past event is to remember the least threatening aspects first, adjust to those, and gradually recall and adjust to the more threatening aspects of the situation. Dreams, which are often filled with symbols or distortions that disguise stressful details, are an example of one such means of dealing adaptively with past stressful events as well as potential future events.

Overcoming Anxiety

Sometimes anxiety is natural and adaptive. When you are facing a forthcoming stressful event, feeling some anxiety is natural, and can be useful in helping you prepare yourself to cope more effectively with the event. Sometimes it is necessary to resolve your feelings about a past stressful event, and mild anxiety from remembering the event is to be expected. On the other hand, anxiety is not normal or adaptive if it interferes with your ability to function effectively day to day, or if it is characterized by a high level of related symptoms.

If anxiety is interfering with your day to day functioning, it is likely that you have let your thinking create an anxiety level that is not normal or adaptive. You can prevent or overcome maladaptive anxiety by undertaking these self-help steps:

1. *Change your beliefs and ways of thinking.* Examine the basis of the threat. Is the threat that lies at the heart of your anxiety more likely (1) a real threat—it has happened or is about to happen, (2) an imagined threat—you think it might happen but there is no evidence yet that it will, or (3) an exaggerated threat—there is a threat, but you misconstrue how threatening it really is?

Most of the time a threat seems real or awful until examined more closely. Irrational ideas or poor thinking can create the illusion of a real threat or exaggerate its magnitude. June created debilitating anxiety by thinking catastrophizing thoughts about how awful it would be to regain weight. Joanne reasoned incorrectly that in order to lose weight she would have to go hungry.

Irrational ideas or thoughts contribute to much maladaptive anxiety. Once you have identified the basis for the felt threat, and the beliefs and ideas that prompt the anxiety, you can take appropriate steps to correct your thinking.

To completely overcome anxiety, you need to change your beliefs and ways of thinking. Gayle had to realize that the meaning she gave to being a beauty queen was the result of falling into certain "thinking traps." She construed the many compliments that people paid her as evidence that she was a sex object, and from this concluded that they did not care about the "real" Gayle.

In fact, Gayle was also quite shy and felt uncomfortable in social situations. Accepting compliments and feeling comfortable in the presence of strangers was difficult for her. She started catastrophizing about how people only liked her because of her looks and how horrible it would be if she weren't beautiful, because no one would like her. In response to the anxiety and fear, she started eating. As she gained weight, people clucked their tongues, and Gayle had more evidence of her worthlessness. The cycle of irrational thoughts continued, producing more weight gain, depression, and anxiety.

By reevaluating the beliefs that give rise to the negative self-talk, and consciously working to reduce negative talk and increase positive self-talk, as discussed in Chapter 4, you can begin to overcome anxiety.

Irrational thoughts and "what if" worries make you feel helpless. When you find yourself worrying about what might happen, turn your focus instead to what you actually can do. Ask yourself what needs to be done to create what you want, and then do it.

If there is nothing you can do, then accept "what is." Worrying does not prevent a feared event from happening. At best, worrying when there is nothing else to do is superstitious; at worst it is debilitating and can even make matters worse. If necessary, expect the worst to happen and plan what to do when it does. This at least gives you some sense of control.

Thought stopping (which was discussed in detail in Chapter 4) is also helpful for managing self-talk and overcoming anxiety. When you find yourself thinking "catastrophizing" thoughts, use thought stopping and turn your thoughts to things that do not produce anxiety. June needed to stop her catastrophizing thoughts about regaining weight and remind herself that she had the ability to manage weight. After all, she was able to teach and motivate others to do so.

If you are exaggerating the potential of a threat, or you are perceiving a threat where none really exists, you need to logically analyze (and if possible empirically test) your beliefs about the threat and the probability of its actually occurring. Upon closer examination, Joanne realized that, in contrast to restrictive dieting, a weight management effort that involved exercise and eating in moderation would make going hungry unnecessary. Although this seemed reasonable, it was not until she actually began losing weight through exercise and moderate eating that she was able to completely overcome her anxiety.

If you are not able to explain why you feel anxious, it is possible you are blocking full awareness of the event from your consciousness, and you need to find a way to bring the source of anxiety to awareness. You may wish to work with a mental health professional, who can use hypnosis, guided imagery, or some other technique to assist you in this regard. Or you may want to try imagery on your own.

2.　*Use imagery to overcome anxiety.* Another technique useful for overcoming anxiety is imagery. (Refer to the instructions given earlier in this chapter for doing imagery.) In your imagination, see the threatening event coming to pass, and the worst possible outcome occurring. Then see yourself coping in the best possible way with that outcome.

Repeat this imagery exercise, varying the scenarios and outcomes, but each time seeing yourself get through it okay. Having acknowledged that the worst could happen but that you would be able to cope effectively with it, you should be better able to keep the anxiety from this threat at a manageable level.

An imagery exercise that may help you involves taking a mental journey in search of something you don't know. Imagine yourself walking through a dark and threatening forest until you encounter a door. Behind that door is something you must confront. You don't know what is behind the door until you open it, and you may feel some fear or concern. Open the door to discover what it is you are seeking. Then after confronting it, walk out of the forest into a sunny meadow where you can relax and recover.

Repeat this trip as many times as necessary until you feel you know the source of your anxiety. Then take appropriate action to deal with the situation. (Even if you think you know the source of your anxiety, doing this imagery exercise can be quite helpful. Sometimes the explanation you have for the problem is not correct, and through imagery you may uncover the true source of your anxiety.)

If you are experiencing anxiety as a result of traumatic memories, you may need professional assistance to deal with them. In order to gain mastery over traumatic memories, you must experience completely the emotions involved, feel that these emotions are valid, forgive yourself for any self-blame, and integrate the memories safely and fully into your consciousness.

3.　*Learn to elicit the relaxation response.* There are many techniques for eliciting the relaxation response—a body state characterized by reduced tension in the muscles, less rapid respiration, decreased oxygen consumption, decreased heart rate, sometimes decreased blood pressure, and increased brain alpha waves.

One of the basic techniques is *deep breathing*. Simply inhale slowly and deeply through your nose and allow your lungs to breathe in as much oxygen as possible. Let your abdomen relax and expand as much as possible, so that you take in as much air as possible. Hold your breath for a few seconds. Then exhale slowly through your mouth, focusing on letting go of muscle tension as you do so, until your lungs feel almost empty. Repeat the cycle several times, until you feel relaxed.

Progressive deep muscle relaxation is helpful for people who may not know how to concentrate on relaxing. It helps you learn the difference between muscle tension and relaxation in three phases: first, tensing a muscle and noticing how it feels; then releasing the tension and paying attention to that feeling; and finally, concentrating on the difference between the two sensations.

To try this, first find a quiet, relaxing place where you will not be disturbed for at least 15 minutes. Then, sit or lie down, removing contact lenses or glasses, and loosening tight clothing.

Start with your hands. Make a fist with one hand and notice how it feels. Your muscles will be taut and strained, maybe even trembling. (Never tense so hard that it hurts.) Hold the tension for a few seconds, then let go. Relax your fist, and let the tension slip away. You may notice that your hand feels lighter or warmer than it did while your muscles were tensed.

Repeat the tensing and relaxing stages one or two times, and notice the difference between the two. Does your hand throb or feel tight when tensed? Does your hand tingle or feel warm when relaxed?

Now progress to the other muscles. Move up the arm to include the forearm, then the whole arm. Completing that arm, do the same sequence—hand, forearm, whole arm—with the other arm. Then focus on your legs, first the feet, then the calves, then the thighs. Continue up the body with the buttocks, abdomen, chest, and shoulders. For your head, tense and relax first the jaw only, then all the facial muscles. Finally, tense and relax the whole body at once, noticing the difference between feeling tense and feeling relaxed.

Once you have completed the entire exercise, allow yourself to enjoy total relaxation for a few minutes before proceeding with your daily activities.

You can also use *imagery* to evoke the relaxation response. Earlier in this chapter you were given detailed instructions for doing imagery. Use your imagination to picture a tranquil setting that has particular appeal to you, perhaps lying on a warm beach feeling the sun on your skin, or standing on a mountain top with the wind in your hair. Take a "mental vacation" for a few minutes whenever you feel the need to relax.

4.   *Learn to clear your mind.* Taking a mental "break" to clear your mind is especially helpful in controlling anxiety that comes from mental agitation and racing thoughts. Sometimes referred to as "meditation," the technique of clearing your mind simply involves concentrating on one pleasant thought, word, or image, and letting the rest of your concerns slip away. June found this quite helpful as a means of quieting her catastrophizing thoughts.

Try to set aside five to ten minutes a day to practice clearing your mind. First, find a place where you are not likely to be disturbed by noise or interruptions. Sit comfortably, loosening any tight clothing and removing contact lenses or glasses. Then, close your eyes and do the deep breathing technique you learned earlier in this chapter.

It helps to focus initially on the feeling of your breath moving in and out. After you begin to feel relaxed with the deep breathing technique, bring to mind something on which you will focus. It may be a single word, such as "one" or "love." Or it may be a thought, such as, "You can do it" or "Be calm, let go." Or it may be a relaxing image, such as a quiet pond or lovely sunset.

If other thoughts intrude while you are trying to concentrate, just let them continue on through your mind and out. Once again bring your attention gently back to your original word, thought, or image.

Do this each time for ten to 20 minutes. When you complete a session, stretch and exhale. With practice, clearing your mind can help you feel refreshed, energetic, and ready to go again.

5.   *Exercise regularly.* In addition to reducing physical arousal, exercise has the further advantage of producing chemical substances in the body that promote calmness and relaxation. Paula used exercise to help her pace the amount of emotion she was able to tolerate as she undertook the work of grieving for her first husband.

Many of the same self-help steps that can help relieve depression can also help relieve ordinary anxiety. These include challenging your perceptions and changing your way of thinking, employing techniques to elicit the relaxation response and to quiet the mind, and engaging in regular exercise. When anxiety is so severe as to be debilitating and prevent day-to-day functioning, the assistance of a mental health professional should also be sought.

Summary

Depression and anxiety are painful emotions that often accompany a weight problem. Whether such emotions actually cause overeating is not clear, but certainly food and eating are used by some sufferers to deal with feelings of depression and anxiety.

For both of these, the way one thinks is a major factor. To overcome these painful emotions it is necessary to challenge and change negative beliefs and self-talk, and to avoid falling into "thinking traps." When either depression or anxiety becomes so severe that one is no longer able to work or enjoy friends, it is time to see a mental health professional for help.

References

1.   Ainsworth, M.D.S., & Bell, S.M. (1969). Some contemporary patterns of mother–infant interaction in the feeding situation. In A. Ambrose (Ed.), *Stimulation in Early Infancy*. New York: Academic Press.

2.   Satter, E.M. (1983). *Child of Mine: Feeding with Love and Good Sense*. Palo Alto, CA: Bull Publishing Company.

3.   Beck, A.T. (1976). *Cognitive Therapy and the Emotional Disorders*. New York: New American Library.

Chapter 8

Managing Anger and Loneliness

NANCY, A SUCCESSFUL *proprietor of her own business and single* parent, was very upset one evening at her weight management group meeting. Recently she had asked her 18-year-old daughter to manage the business for her for one week so that she could go on a long-delayed and much-needed vacation. When the daughter not only refused but moved out to go live with her father, Nancy was both hurt and terribly angry.

Bitterly she blamed herself for being too indulgent and allowing her daughter to become lazy and insensitive. When she told her group that she planned to refuse to pay her daughter's car insurance or education expenses, she was astounded and further angered that the group members did not endorse her actions nor sympathize with her situation in the way she had expected.

"You don't understand," she said, "I've never asked her to do anything for me before. This is the first time. I've been sick. She can see that I need a vacation. I've been good to her and taken care of her all her life, and just this once I asked for something from her and she ran out on me. I place a high value on family. Family should stick together and be there for each other. You can't believe how hurt I am. It's more than I can bear. Things are so awful that I don't see how I can give any concern to weight management at this time. I don't see any point in continuing to come to this group."

Like Nancy, Carla impressed people with her apparent personal power and competence. She had been an assistant bank vice president before returning to school at age 35 to finish her bachelor's degree, and at school she got only the highest marks. At about the same time that she returned to school, she also entered an intimate living together relationship with a man who was a professor at the university she was attending. She completed her undergraduate degree with a 4.0 average, and planned to go on to a masters in business administration. She applied to two very prominent business schools.

Carla had always fought a weight problem, and the stress of maintaining high grades and coping with a change in lifestyle produced increased emotional eating, a reduction in regular exercise, and a gradual weight gain. As her weight continued to climb, her lover became increasingly critical of her weight and her eating habits.

When she was rejected by both business schools of her choice, Carla was greatly disappointed. Her eating habits worsened, as did her relationship. The more her lover criticized her, the more she demanded that he accept her as she was. As her anger increased, her eating habits became even worse, and she gained more weight.

Molly was a buyer in the high fashion department of a large department store. Although she loved her job, she had difficulty tolerating the regular interruptions and petty problems brought to her by both her boss and her staff. It never seemed to fail that whenever she was in the middle of a report, someone suddenly needed her immediate attention.

Sometimes she would stifle the angry feelings that would overcome her when she was needlessly interrupted; at other times she would make a sarcastic remark intended to communicate to the other person her anger at the imposition. Feeling constantly frustrated and hassled, she would soothe herself by munching on the candy bars she kept in her desk drawer. As a result, her weight kept creeping up, and her professional image was being threatened.

The Determinants of Anger

People who are prone to anger and are without effective coping strategies are likely to suffer health impairments, diminished work efficiency, and disruption of personal relationships. For Nancy, Carla, and Molly, anger made weight management more difficult. To increase their chances for life-long success with weight management, they needed to better understand what anger is and what prompts it, and learn to cope with it more effectively.

Anger is an important emotion that can enable people to function effectively in life. It is a signal emotion that tells you your rights are being trampled, that your needs are not being met, and that something needs to change. Used adaptively, anger can make life better. Handled inappropriately—when it is either held in or let out at the wrong time—anger can cause problems in life.

Anger results when there is a gap between what you want and what you get. When your expectations are not met, or someone commits a transgression of the "rules," as was the case with Nancy, you are likely to react with anger. When you are frustrated in your attempt to attain some goal, when you feel rejected or unfairly treated, when there is a threat to your sense of self-worth, or when you are ridiculed or put down, as happened to Carla, anger can build and may become internalized. When things don't go the way you want them to or think they should, as with Molly, anger may become a continuing problem.

Anger can be the result of actual injury, or simply your belief that you have been or may be injured. Anger is an attempt to gain control over a situation or to get agreement about your being "right" about something.

Anger can range in intensity from mere annoyance to furious rage, depending on the circumstances and the view you take of them. When you are merely annoyed or irritated, you may feel some minor muscle tension. The more angry you are, the higher the level of physical arousal is likely to be. Your face may flush, your heart rate increase, and breathing accelerate. In its more intense stages, anger may be felt like a wave of heat rolling over you.

When angry, you may become aggressive toward someone, verbally attacking the person with insults or sarcasm or even actually striking him. Or you may displace your aggressive feelings onto someone or something else, throw a temper tantrum, or take some passive aggressive action—slamming doors or kicking a piece of furniture. Alternatively, you may simply withdraw into an angry silence.

Although anger seems to come from some provocative event—real, imagined, remembered, or anticipated—it is really your interpretation and evaluation of the event that gives rise to anger. The event merely triggers the thinking process which in turn determines the anger. The Stoic philosopher, Epictetus, once said, "Men are disturbed not by things, but by the view they take of them."

The particular life philosophy you hold—i.e., the sum of your beliefs, values, attitudes, and rules—is a major determinant of the meaning you give to an event.[1] Your life philosophy in effect creates a filter through which you relate to the world. It causes you to look for and selectively attend to information to support your point of view. In this way it colors your evaluation of events. And you keep emotionally loaded past events "alive," and anticipated future happenings vivid by remembering or dwelling on them.

How you react to an event once you feel angry will depend on a number of factors. If you think showing anger might change things, you are likely to exhibit some kind of behavior that expresses anger. Nancy let her daughter know clearly how hurt and angry she felt, and she threatened to retaliate by cutting off economic support.

Responding aggressively, however, often increases your anger. Acting aggressively tends to reinforce your belief that you are justified in being angry. If your anger doesn't work to get the other person to change, you may become even more angry.

On the other hand, if you think showing anger or acting aggressively will hurt your position or incur some cost to you, or if you believe that showing anger is not appropriate, you may refrain from expressing anger openly, though you may express it in other ways. Carla wasn't able to show her anger, partly because she wasn't sure with whom she was angry, but it found expression in secret binge eating.

But even expressing anger appropriately doesn't completely eliminate the problem. Although Molly periodically let others know she was angry with them, she also used food to cope with the physical arousal that is always a part of feeling angry.

"Angry" Philosophies

Anger is always created and maintained by the way in which you think—by the ideas, beliefs, perceptions, and attitudes you hold. The more anger-provoking ideas you have, the more prone you are to being angry and acting aggressively. Your "life philosophy"—the point of view you take—influences whether and to what degree you experience anger.

Depending on your life philosophy, you are likely to be overly sensitive to elements of injustice or signs of hassle in situations. You may attribute the actions of others to hostile motivations, or you may habitually take things too personally. You can re-anger yourself by remembering (perhaps becoming obsessed about) past slights, and you may overreact to minor frustrations.

In a very real sense, your thinking is thus "programmed" to create anger. Certain groups of ideas or beliefs form the core of specific "angry" philosophies and produce different types of anger.

Self-Centered Anger

Self-centered anger is "I" centered. It springs from the idea that because "I" do not personally like something or do not want something to happen, or "I" find someone's behavior undesirable or even obnoxious, it should not happen, or the person must not behave that way. A person who is used to being in control, used to being the authority, or not used to having her views challenged is often prone to self-centered anger. The assumption is made that if "I" deem an action or event wrong, based on whatever standards "I" choose, that it *should not/must not* occur.

When something happens that is unfortunate, inconvenient, deplorable, dangerous, etc., the self-centered angry person concludes it is so awful as to be virtually unbearable. She will almost certainly become outraged and probably act in some revengeful way. She condemns either the world for letting it happen or the offensive person for doing such a thing. Not only are the offending person's acts bad, but he too is bad and should be severely punished. Nancy's anger was self-centered anger.

Impersonal Anger

Impersonal anger is a variation of self-centered anger. At its core are the three assumptions that characterize self-centered anger: l) that an action or event that is deemed wrong should not and must not occur, 2) that when the event or act does occur it is awful and unbearable, and 3) that not only is what happened "rotten," but so is the person who perpetrated the offending action.

Rather than relying on personal rules, however, the person experiencing impersonal anger invokes an explicit or implicit code of rules that pertains to some community. (Examples of explicit rules are constitutions, treaties, laws, ordinances, contracts, and agreements. Implicit rules include social taboos and cultural norms.)

Becoming angry with a neighbor for violating a community leash law and allowing her dog to run into your yard invokes an explicit code of rules. Becoming outraged upon hearing of a child who was sexually molested by a parent invokes an implicit code of conduct. Nancy became angry with her weight management group, because she felt they violated an implicit rule that group members should be sympathetic to each other's problems.

Whether self-centered anger or impersonal anger, the core ideas are that it is right and proper to demand that another be held to a certain standards of behavior, and that it is legitimate to condemn and even punish another if he or she violates such standards.

Self-Worth Anger

Self-worth is another theme that can be central to the experience of anger— a perceived threat to one's sense of being worthwhile. The person who is caught up in self-worth anger believes that her self-worth depends on what others think of her, and on how well she does in gaining the acknowledgement, acceptance, and love of others.

The person prone to self-worth anger is unduly concerned about what others think. She often sets high, perfectionistic standards for herself. She feels she must do well and win approval, especially from those she deems significant, or else she is worthless.

When others don't treat her well or are overtly rejecting or critical, she interprets this as evidence of her lack of worth, rather than as evidence of their shortcomings. When they do acknowledge and accept her, she is likely to either discount such approval, or else be resentful that she had to "work so hard" to earn it. She tends to turn anger inward to herself, rather than directing it outward to the critical or rejecting source.

On a conscious level, the person experiencing self-worth anger may be quite critical of herself and others, often engaging in "shoulding" and condemning. At a less conscious level, however, she tends to generalize from the undesirable actions of others to her own self-worth.

Sometimes she exhibits "defensive high self-esteem." That is, she seems to have a healthy sense of self-worth. She may have been successful in getting people to approve of her, and when they are, her self-esteem is temporarily high. But her sense of self-worth is fragile because it is dependent on the continued good grace of others. Prolonged or frequent assaults can easily shatter her facade, resulting in a deepening of anger and/or more depression and lowered self-esteem.

Carla was the victim of self-worth anger. Her sense of self-worth depended on what others thought of her. Although her professors rewarded her efforts in school with praise and high grades, she was constantly criticized at home for her weight and her eating habits. Periodically she protested that her lover should accept her as she was, but she secretly believed that she should be able to control her eating and her weight, and when she could not, she berated herself.

Unhappily, she believed that his condemnations were justified. With the continued onslaught of criticism, her self-esteem declined and the anger within her grew. When she was rejected by both business schools to which she had applied, her self-worth received yet another blow. Instead of blaming unjust admission standards or political considerations, she took the rejection personally. Her eating habits further deteriorated, and eating became a self-destructive expression of anger directed inward.

Low Frustration Tolerance Anger

Molly is an example of the person prone to low frustration tolerance anger. Her tolerance for interruptions was minimal. At the core of her life philosophy were beliefs about how the world should be arranged so that she could get pretty much what she wanted, when she wanted it, and without too much hassle. When things didn't go smoothly according to the way she thought they should, or when she felt thwarted or presented with difficult circumstances, she overreacted with frustration and anger. She wanted things to be easy, smooth, and hassle-free.

When it isn't that way, it is "too much to bear" and "shouldn't be this way." Someone else (or the world) is blamed. The felt anger is essentially a scream of outrage against any interruption of the smooth flow of events. To quiet the arousal that accompanies the outrage, Molly eats.

What Alters the Experience of Anger

Many things can influence or alter your experience of anger. Your anger is likely to be more intense if you believe someone intentionally has tried to hurt you, or if you feel the motivation of your aggressor has been arbitrary, unjustified, or selfish. Nancy's anger was strong, and she planned to retaliate against her daughter because she felt that the daughter's actions had been intentionally hurtful, unjustified, and selfish. If you think your anger is justified, as Nancy did, you are likely to experience more intense anger.

Your anger is likely to be less intense, however, if you feel you have some choice in the situation. That is, feeling that you can control or cope more effectively with a situation that tends to provoke anger diminishes its intensity. When Molly got her co-workers to agree to the circumstances under which she should be interrupted, and was able to set aside some "do not interrupt time" for herself, she made some progress in coping with anger.

Discovering a different explanation for a provoking event can change anger. When Nancy learned that her daughter's actions were prompted by fear that she would never be able to measure up to her mother's high standards, and that she was likely to do something wrong in the business while her mother was on vacation, a new light was cast on the matter.

Likewise, giving a different meaning to an event can change anger. Once Carla was able to reinterpret the business school rejections as failings of the selection committees of the schools, rather than as evidence of her lack of worth, she felt somewhat better.

Your physical condition may also influence how prone you are to anger at any given time. Hunger, fatigue, hormones, and other biochemical factors may play a role at times in lowering the threshold at which an event elicits anger. Some research has demonstrated, for example, that anger is more likely to occur just before dinner.

Restrictive diets which make you hungry may make anger more likely by making you more sensitive to provocations. The pressure to reduce the accompanying physical arousal then leads to breaking the diet, and this in turn produces anger directed at the self for falling short of perfectionistic dieting standards.

Healthy and Unhealthy Anger

Adopting a set of beliefs, ideas, and attitudes (life philosophy) is necessary in order to make decisions in life. Since anger, as well as other emotions, is rooted in the particular set of beliefs (i.e., life philosophy) you adopt, it is not possible (nor especially desirable) to completely eliminate the experience of anger. It is possible, however, to reduce the probability of experiencing anger that does not serve you, and to minimize minor annoyances and irritations.

To do this you must first recognize how your particular life philosophy creates your emotions. When you hold strong "should" beliefs that get rigidly applied to yourself and others, you are usually setting yourself up for anger. If you can let go of some of these "shoulds" and be more accepting of yourself and others, you are likely to experience less anger.

The challenge is to differentiate between healthy anger and unhealthy anger. Healthy anger serves you and helps you get what you want and need. Unhealthy anger prevents you from getting what you want or need in the long-run. It usually interferes with relationships and ultimately makes your experience of life unsatisfactory.

To distinguish healthy anger, it is helpful to consider the basic values that all humans hold. Among these are staying alive, living happily or with an acceptable amount of pleasure and a minimum of pain, living comfortably in a social group or community in which one is basically accepted, and relating intimately and lovingly with one or a selected few people. Healthy anger leads to the realization of these basic human values or goals, while unhealthy anger thwarts your ability to achieve them.

When anger occurs, there are both rational and irrational thoughts or ideas that lie behind and prompt the anger. (Irrational beliefs are discussed in detail in Chapter 3.) Rational thoughts or ideas can assist you to realize your basic goals. Irrational thoughts can lead you to behave in ways that undermine your goals.

Nancy's anger came largely from irrational ideas about how her daughter should act. The anger these notions produced prompted her to consider retaliating against her. Had she done so, she would have further driven a wedge between herself and her daughter and undermined one of Nancy's basic goals—to relate lovingly with her family.

Eventually she was able to accept that her daughter needed to assert her own independence and had a right to refuse the responsibility her mother wanted her to assume. By accepting her daughter's rights to independence and to refuse requests, even requests from her mother, Nancy opened the way for a dialogue between herself and her daughter that could facilitate the realization of her basic goals.

Carla's anger undermined her ability to achieve the basic human values because she placed too much emphasis on other people's evaluations of her, and because she was caught in the "thinking trap" of perfectionism. She needed to replace the irrational ideas—that it was necessary for her happiness that everyone think highly of her, and that she always be perfect—with the rational ideas that while it is nice to be loved and appreciated by others, that is not always possible, and doing your best is more important than striving for perfection.

Likewise, Molly had to give up irrational ideas about the way the world and her life should function, and replace them with a more rational and realistic picture of the way her job was set up to work. While she was able to gain some measure of control by rearranging certain aspects of the job, she had chosen to be in a job that by definition involved working closely with other people. By changing her point of view, Molly's perception of her job, her relationships, and herself all changed.

Overcoming Anger

There are a number of things you can do to avoid unhealthy anger or to overcome and cope more effectively with anger when it does occur.[2]

1.   *Learn to tell the difference between healthy and unhealthy anger.* Learn to identify the irrational thoughts and ideas that prompt anger, and replace them with more rational thoughts and ideas that facilitate your achieving the things that are most important to your happiness.

One way to learn how to tell the difference between healthy and unhealthy anger is to keep a journal of your anger experiences, including the lesser experiences of annoyance and irritation. Record what the circumstances were that prompted you to feel angry. Note especially the beliefs or ideas you hold that are at the bottom of the anger. These can easily be identified because they usually contain the words "should" or "shouldn't."

If you are "shoulding," you are probably also blaming someone, perhaps yourself. These are the ideas and reactions you must change. Look for a different interpretation and another way of viewing the situation. In the end, you may simply have to acknowledge that you don't like the situation, but that allowing yourself to stay angry about it is not likely to change things, nor will it do you any good.

2.   *Choose carefully the issues on which you will take a stand.* People who are prone to anger often attach too much importance to events around them. Rather than choosing when to take a stand, they react indiscriminately to many events, including those quite distant from themselves. And they often take things personally.

In fact, there may be times when anger is appropriate and healthy. The question to answer first is, "Will being angry aid the realization of the things that are most important to me?" Be careful. Irrational thoughts and ideas may be lurking in the disguise of concern for basic human values. Nancy initially tried to claim that she was angry with her daughter because she valued highly having a loving family, and that her daughter was thwarting the realization of that value. In fact, Nancy held a number of beliefs about how people, including her daughter, should and should not act.

3.   *Acknowledge unhealthy anger and assume full responsibility for it.* When you find yourself blaming or condemning others, stop and ask yourself how you contributed to the situation's turning out as it did. But don't fall into the trap of automatically blaming yourself. Just consider as objectively and dispassionately as possible what things you did or didn't do that allowed the situation to occur. Look for and find the anger-instigating thoughts and ideas that prompted the unhealthy anger. Then decide what action you need to take or ideas you need to adopt in order to realize your basic goals.

4. *Express anger appropriately.* Avoid indiscriminately venting anger, because it reinforces the belief that anger is both unavoidable and acceptable. Contrary to some beliefs, anger is not a primitive or unavoidable drive over which you have no control. By giving free expression to anger you simply rehearse the anger-producing thoughts and ideas, which further engrains them and abets anger.

On the other hand, don't squelch or deny anger. Learn to express it appropriately and objectively. Before expressing anger, it helps to pause and take several deep breaths. You may even need to take a walk and collect your thoughts, or wait a day or two before dealing with the situation. Just be sure that you do not simply deny or stuff it down, as Carla did. And when you do express how you feel, avoid blaming, and take responsibility for your experience. "When you do such-and-such, I feel such-and-such," rather than "You make me . . ."

5. *Learn to identify the cues that anger is imminent.* By keeping a record of your experience of anger, you will learn to recognize the various external and internal cues that signal its onset. There may be certain situations that always prompt anger for you. (Being interrupted was one for Molly.) Often drinking too much alcohol will allow anger to surface too easily, or at least make you more vulnerable to anger-provoking situations. Having identified those situations in which anger is more likely to occur, you may be able to avoid them in the future, or at least plan a different way to respond.

Become more aware of the physical cues that indicate your anger is rising. These may include a change in the tone or volume of your voice, a hot flush in your face, or a tensing of some muscle groups. Use these cues as signals to relax, take several deep breaths, and change your behavior.

Learn to identify the ways in which you behave that act as provocation to others. These might include making threatening gestures, cutting others off, making threats, teasing, covertly sabotaging another, refusing to listen to another's point of view, or verbally abusing someone—calling them names or hurling epithets at them. You must be willing to change such behaviors, and become more conciliatory and friendly in these situations.

6. *Prepare for a potentially provocative situation.* When you know that a potentially provocative situation is in the offing, prepare for it by using stress-inoculation. (Using stress inoculation is discussed in Chapter 4.) Nancy used this technique to prepare herself for the telephone call she planned to make to her daughter, inviting her to come home for the holidays.

7. *Use relaxation techniques to release muscle tension and deal with the physical arousal of anger.* In the previous chapter in the section on overcoming anxiety, eliciting the relaxation response was discussed. (Other techniques for relaxing and managing anger are given by McKay, et. al. in

When Anger Hurts.[3]) Learn to take a couple of deep breaths and mentally tell yourself to relax and stay centered in the face of anger.

Take a "time out" to get your emotions under control. Additional suggestions for dealing with the arousal of anger and achieving relaxation are to get some exercise, take a long, hot bath, get a massage, use imagery, and listen to soothing music.

8. ***Use distraction techniques to better manage the physical arousal of anger.*** When you are feeling angry or upset, your body reacts. You may feel increasing tension—perhaps a knot in your stomach, neck, or jaw. You may start to shake or your tone of voice may change. To say in control, you need to be able to manage the physical arousal that comes with feeling angry. It helps to distract your attention from the upsetting situation and to focus on relaxing and letting go. You can accomplish this by counting backwards, using thought stopping, or engaging in pleasant imagery.

9. ***Develop better communication skills.*** Having good communication skills is vital for being able to express anger appropriately. Learn to be assertive, rather than aggressive or passive. Chapter 6, *Improving Your Relationships*, focuses on this, as well as on how to manage conflict more effectively.

Expressing Justified Anger

For some people, the difficulty is not controlling anger, but accepting that they are angry and knowing what to do about it. Women, in particular, have difficulty owning and expressing anger.

Some may believe that good, loving people don't get angry, or that they have no right to be angry. They fear they may be rejected if they are openly angry. Others grew up in families where emotional expression was discouraged, or only parents had the privilege of displaying their feelings. Or for still others, anger may feel so overwhelming that they fear losing control if they even acknowledge their anger. When justified anger is not owned and expressed, the person who has it may use food, alcohol, drugs, sex, or any number of other things, to try to deaden their feelings.

There are times when anger is justified, and needs to be owned and expressed appropriately. This is particularly true if you have been emotionally, physically, or sexually abused.

Some people believe that the remedy for such experiences is to forgive and forget. Dr. Susan Forward, a psychotherapist and incest survivor who has written extensively on the subject, argues that forgiveness is a trap. First, the victim must own and express her anger and pain, though not necessarily directly to the perpetrator, in order to set herself free. Forgiveness, if it comes, is later. The real work of healing abuse involves grieving for the tremendous losses incurred—of childhood, of innocence, of trust, of safety, of nurturing and respectful parents—and taking back power over your life.

Concluding Thoughts About Anger

Anger is the least well understood of the emotions. As with other emotions, however, it is largely caused by your beliefs and ways of thinking. Although it is probably not possible to remove all sources of irritation and annoyance, the experience of unhealthy anger can largely be eliminated, and the upset from anger reduced by changing beliefs and ways of thinking.

Some other important steps include choosing when to get angry, expressing anger appropriately, learning to identify and respond to the cues of anger, preparing for provocation, using relaxation techniques, using distraction techniques, and developing better communication skills. In cases of abuse, anger is justified, and needs to be owned and expressed, to take back power over your life.

Loneliness

Everyone experiences occasional feelings of separateness from others, feelings of alienation, social awkwardness, or periodic disappointment because there is no one with whom to share some activity. For some people the pain of loneliness is more severe. When loneliness persists, it can lead to emotional disorders and impaired physical health.

Unwanted isolation is distressing, and is often accompanied by feelings of sadness, anxiety, anger, self-deprecation, boredom, low self-esteem, and depression. People who are lonely may abuse alcohol, use drugs, or even turn to suicide for relief. Some people turn to food to alleviate loneliness, only to end up feeling worse, as the resulting obesity contributes further to their isolation.

Loneliness is not simply being alone. Indeed, some people enjoy being alone and choose to avoid much social contact. Loneliness comes when a person wants the experience of human relatedness, but it is not forthcoming.

Feeling lonely can be the result of having too few social companions or people to go to for emotional support. It arises from the repeated disappointment of having to forego activities that depend upon the participation of another person, or having to participate alone in activities that are usually shared by others. In other cases, the lonely person has other people in her life, but is unable to reach out to them or relate in an intimate and meaningful way.

Just being with others does not necessarily prevent loneliness. Some "empty shell" marriages actually promote loneliness, as the partners share little of each other's lives. Loneliness results when a person feels estranged from, misunderstood, or rejected by others. For some people a disturbing and persistent sense of separateness from others is the core of loneliness. Loneliness is having no one with whom you can share hopes, joys, fears, and disappointments.

While for most people loneliness may come from too few social ties, it can also be the result of having unrealistic expectations. Some people want more closeness, more one-to-one interaction, more commitment, or more of some other quality than the other person in the relationship can provide.

In many cases, the lonely person chooses the "wrong" person with whom to pursue a close and intimate relationship. A person who is not available because he is in another committed relationship, or who is primarily interested in getting his own needs met, is a poor choice for the investment of relationship time and energy.

Sometimes a lonely person does have friends, or even intimate relationships, but her expectations for what these relationships can do for her are unrealistic. She may want the other person to always be there for her when she wants him, or to know her every wish and desire without her having to mention it. Her disappointment when her needs are not met may leave her feeling alone, unloved, and—when the other person gets upset at such unreasonable demands—misunderstood.

To avoid loneliness, people need to have a sense of social integration, and they need to have opportunities for emotional intimacy. Ties to a social group, such as a network of friends, a club, a neighborhood organization can provide the sense of social connectedness.

Having a spouse or intimate partner provides the opportunity for emotional intimacy. Losing either can cause loneliness. This is why someone who has lots of friends but no one lover can feel lonely, and conversely, why someone who has a lover but no other friends can also be lonely.

A survey by the Institute for Social Research showed that one in six Americans does not have a friend to whom they can confide personal problems. In other research 19% of respondents reported that they did not have "many very good friends." A nationwide 1983 Louis Harris poll found that 16% of people interviewed reported socializing with others only two or three times a month or less. Clearly, loneliness is a problem for a significant number of people.

Social bonds have long been considered essential to psychological well-being, and it has been shown that those who lack others to turn to for emotional support (or who experience loneliness despite having a social network) are prone to stress-related illnesses and psychiatric disorders. Deficient social relations and social isolation have been linked to increased mortality as well as mental and physical problems. The extent to which loneliness contributes to the development and maintenance of obesity has not been studied, but clinical experience suggests that loneliness can be a factor that makes successful weight management more difficult.

Joanne was a single parent of two sons, ages 12 and 15. She returned to the university at age 40 to pursue a master's degree. As a result, she left the friends who had supported her through the divorce and moved to a college community some distance away. As an older women in a highly competitive graduate program, she focused her energies on her school work and her sons, and over the course of a year gained 40 pounds. Relating to the other students in her program was difficult; they tended to be much younger, and Joanne felt that they did not want to make friends with her because they felt there was little in common to share.

The only fellow student Joanne did attempt to befriend, she ultimately rejected as "too into herself." As for her neighbors and other members of the local community, Joanne dismissed them as "too linear," and not willing or able to share her interests. Revisiting her old friends was difficult because they were so far away, and Joanne didn't want them to see her having gained so much weight. Indeed, she feared they might criticize her, as her long-time hairdresser had done when he told her she looked disgusting with all that weight.

Ida spent most of her time watching TV, sleeping, or eating. She had always been shy; reaching out and making friends was very painful. She never knew what to say, and she felt uncomfortable in groups. Because she only had a part-time job, she had little money to go places or do things, and she had no one to do things with anyway.

Her mother lived some distance away, but if she needed something, Ida hurried to do her bidding. As long as Ida complied with her mother's wishes, nothing was said about her weight, but on those occasions when her mother got upset, Ida was sure to be harangued about how slovenly and lazy she was.

At well over 280 pounds, Jody had been a very vocal member of a fat-liberation, fat-is-beautiful group, until she decided that the other members of the group weren't as dedicated as she was to the cause. She took up the campaign against the social ostracism of fat people on her own.

She changed her name so that it more clearly signified her willingness to go it alone, and she spent her energies speaking to groups and making media appearances to protest discrimination against fat people, and what she perceived as unethical and harmful treatment. She freely admitted that she trusted no one, not even other fat people. Her defiant demeanor denied her obvious aloneness.

These three women demonstrate what the research on loneliness indicates about who gets lonely and why. Lonely people generally have greater difficulty making social contacts and maintaining social relationships. They feel uncomfortable introducing themselves, initiating social contacts, or asserting themselves.

They have difficulty taking social risks, participating in groups, or enjoying themselves at social gatherings. Sharing their opinions or ideas with others is something they find hard to do, and they tend to be less responsive to attempts at social contact made by others. Often they approach social encounters with cynicism and mistrust.

They tend to evaluate themselves critically, and they expect others to reject them. They tend to rate others negatively and critically as well, possibly demonstrating a pattern of "rejecting others first." And they express less desire for continued contact than do socially integrated people.

Some people with weight problems tend to be introverted, to avoid others, and not be tuned into reality. Even when such people have access to a social network, they are not likely to make use of it. It's as if they are resigned to further loneliness, and engage in passive, ineffective coping responses, such as watching TV, overeating, taking tranquilizers, oversleeping, or overworking.

These reactions may be part of an effort to protect fragile self-esteem. Loneliness is associated with feelings of low self-worth, self-consciousness in social interaction, and self-blame for social failures. As with Joanne, Ida, and Jody, lonely people may be attempting to minimize risk of negative feedback from others, by either withdrawing, complying excessively with the wishes of others, or rebelling.

By withdrawing, Joanne effectively eliminated threats of criticism or rejection. She defined her fellow students and her fellow community members as "not her kind of people," and consequently closed off the possibility of social interaction that might alleviate loneliness. She refused to visit her old friends out of fear of criticism of her weight. Not only did she close herself off from the possibility of friends who could support her, with no spouse she had no attachment figure to provide emotional intimacy. Her only source for this was her two sons.

She buried herself in her work as a means of escape and in a desperate attempt to bolster sinking self-esteem. Although she held forth that she was proud of her accomplishments, in fact she was secretly extremely self-critical.

Ida's excessive compliance with her mother's wishes is an example of the kind of effort that many overweight people make in a vain attempt to avoid criticism and social rejection. In addition, Ida had never learned how to make friends. Her parents, especially her mother, had always been critical of her childhood friends, so Ida had rarely developed friendships even as a child. She didn't know what to say to others, and it was always easier to be alone. Ida's mother was a woman who always kept to herself, and Ida learned to do so, too. The only significant interaction Ida had was with her mother, who held power over her with the threat of criticism and rejection.

By choosing rebellion as her strategy, Jody managed to invalidate sources of negative feedback. She was suspicious and distrustful of others, and she never let anyone get close to her. She blamed her parents for her weight because they had forced her to go on diets and take pills as a youngster. She blamed the health professions for keeping fat people fat by putting them on diets, treating them as problems, and not responding to them as "normal" people. Being intelligent and articulate, she was able to quote statistics and distort facts about obesity to bolster her point of view, and to deny information that might challenge her contention that severe over-fatness should be acceptable to others as well as to the person affected by it.

While Jody's rebellion was overt, in fact rebelling is more often an internal experience. Some obese people secretly rage at the ridicule, criticism, and discrimination to which they are often subjected. As a result, they bring an attitude of cynicism and mistrust to all social contacts, and this is communicated nonverbally. An "invisible barrier" is erected, that effectively prohibits the development of intimate relationships.

Withdrawal, compliance, and rebellion do not enhance self-esteem; they serve to protect an already fragile self-concept from further negative feedback. They also foster the persistence of loneliness, create fertile ground for depression and anger, and mediate against successful weight reduction.

More effective strategies are needed to relieve loneliness, to cope more effectively with unavoidable loneliness, and to prevent loneliness if possible.

Strategies for Relieving Loneliness

Loneliness originates from the way people think and behave. In addition, certain situations foster loneliness. A wide variety of strategies for dealing with loneliness are needed.

Some person-oriented strategies include social skills training and changing beliefs and thinking. Situation-oriented strategies include restructuring the existing social or physical environment, and finding ways to increase the number of social opportunities.

Improving Social Skills

Chapter 6, *Improving Your Relationships,* deals more specifically with the behaviors needed to create better relationships with others, including how to communicate more effectively and assertively. Among the social skills that may need attention are how to initiate social contacts, how to overcome shyness, and how to achieve intimacy in a relationship. Of particular importance for people with a weight problem is learning to deal more effectively with criticism and conflict.

Loneliness is the product of withdrawing from people, often as a protection from criticism and rejection. To overcome loneliness, you must be willing to take chances, to be vulnerable to possible criticism and rejection, and to reach out to others.

Check in your community for programs that give social skills training. Such programs usually use techniques such as modeling, role playing, performance feedback with videotape, and homework assignments that can be of great assistance in improving your ability to relate better to others. Check with your community mental health department, departments of psychology or counseling in local colleges and universities, or the psychological referral service that is listed in the phone book for such programs.

Changing Beliefs and Thinking

Lonely people are usually plagued by thoughts that create feelings of anxiety and paralyze their ability to engage in effective social contacts.

"I don't know what to do. I'll just make a fool of myself if I try."

"I know they think I'm fat and disgusting."

"I bet they don't like having me around."

"I'm sure she feels we don't have anything in common."

These are the kind of self-defeating thoughts that seem to come automatically into the heads of lonely people. From Chapter 3 you learned that certain beliefs and thinking traps cause these kinds of thoughts. Decisions you made about yourself and your worthiness, unrealistically high standards you may have set for yourself, making a decision based on one incident from the past, and jumping to conclusions are just some of the beliefs or thinking traps that produce such thoughts.

In Chapter 4 you learned to use the "double column" technique to identify negative self-talk and create competing arguments. Use this technique again now to identify the automatic thoughts you have about yourself and others when it comes to being involved in social contacts.

Use the form provided on page 174 (sample on page 173), or make your own. Draw a line down the center of a page to make two columns. Label the left column "Automatic Thoughts," and the right column "Rebuttals." In the left column write the automatic, negative thoughts that keep you from reaching out to others. Then use the right-hand column to create a more rational, realistic thought that you can use in rebuttal of the negative, automatic thoughts that keep you stuck.

Restructuring the Existing Environment

Having adequate social skills and being able to think "smart" are strategies that can help to remove or at least reduce sources of loneliness; but sometimes you must alter the situation.

Because Joanne was so involved with her work, she had little time to pursue friendships. To some degree she was a mismatch in her social environment at school—most students were much younger than she was and didn't have two sons to support. Her old network of friends was some distance away, and even if she had wanted to see them, making contact would have been difficult. Ida's isolation was in part reinforced by her economic circumstances—she had only a part-time job and little money with which to get involved in other activities.

Time, distance, money, and match with the social environment are all

sample *Challenging Negative Thoughts*

Automatic Thoughts Thoughts that keep you from reaching out to others	*Rebuttals* Thoughts that can help you to reach out to others
1) I'm different than they are and I don't belong.	1) When I feel like an outsider, it's because I'm judging myself. I need to make a special effort to make contact.
2) I'd rather be by myself; I prefer my own company.	2) It's good to enjoy being by myself sometimes, but having friends is important too. To have a friend I have to reach out and be a friend.
3) We have nothing in common, so why should I bother to have a conversation with her? She'll just think I'm dumb.	3) I won't know if we have anything in common unless we talk. Maybe I should give both of us a chance.

Challenging Negative Thoughts

Automatic Thoughts	**Rebuttals**
Thoughts that keep you from reaching out to others	*Thoughts that can help you to reach out to others*

situational factors that mediate against a solution to loneliness. Even so, it is possible to find ways to change the existing environment to improve chances of a solution and encourage social contact.

Sandy accepted a job in a large organization. She soon discovered that most people in the organization kept to themselves; there was little or no socializing outside of that necessary for the job. Dissatisfied with the unfriendly atmosphere, her first step was to place a notice in the organization's newsletter to organize a network of people who would like to have someone else with whom to share lunch. Next, she spoke with the boss of her department and convinced him to arrange for the entire department to go out to lunch once a month. Her efforts helped create a friendlier atmosphere and reduced Sandy's sense of social isolation at work.

Sandy was creative in finding a way to change a needlessly alienating environment and foster a friendlier atmosphere at her place of work. There are many ways to increase opportunities for social contact. Joining or forming a group of people whose purpose is to work together to accomplish a shared goal is another way.

When it is not possible to change an existing environment, it may be necessary to leave it and seek one that is more supportive.

Learning to Cope With Unavoidable Loneliness

Sometimes loneliness cannot be avoided. People who divorce or suffer the death of a loved one must learn how to cope with the unavoidable loneliness that such situations are likely to cause—at least for a while. When better coping skills are brought to bear upon this kind of "transitional" loneliness, adjustment takes place more rapidly and painful emotions are minimized. It is particularly helpful for divorced or separated people to join a group of other people dealing with the same problem.

Family and friends are important for emotional support during bereavement. It may also be helpful to seek the support of a mental health professional to facilitate the grieving process. The bereaved person should also find an interest or project which she can devote her energies to—perhaps becoming a volunteer in an organization she admires.

When loneliness cannot be avoided, it is crucial to develop aloneness skills. While many people come to enjoy and even treasure time alone, others, especially those who have spent most of their life in a close relationship with another, can find being alone threatening and painful.

In almost every life there comes a time when being alone is a necessity, and learning how to enjoy it is important. Developing hobbies you can do alone, enjoying reading or finding other solitary pursuits is part of learning how to be alone.

Preventing Loneliness

It is probably not possible to prevent loneliness entirely, but it is possible to prevent unnecessary loneliness. Prevention starts by identifying who is at high risk of suffering loneliness. Such people include women, the young, the unmarried, the unemployed, low-income people, the elderly, the handicapped, the mentally ill, the severely obese, and caretakers of chronically disabled or ill people. If you are one of these, or if you know someone who falls into one of these categories, be especially aware that loneliness may be a problem. Be alert to how you might help prevent or relieve it.

One solution that has received some widespread publicity recently is having a pet to care for. Dogs, cats and other pets provide a source of unconditional love. They give their owners an opportunity to provide and care for a living thing that needs attention. Research has shown that people with pets function better than those without.

Unnecessary loneliness is less likely when the family interaction is healthy. It is in the family that children learn how to interact with others and develop a sense of self-esteem. They learn how to interact socially by observing how their parents interact socially.

Parents who are socially withdrawn and anxious tend to rear children who are similarly withdrawn and anxious. Parents who exhibit cynicism and mistrust teach children to do the same. Likewise, parents who are overprotective, critical, or rejecting toward their children sow the seeds of low self-esteem that can lead ultimately to loneliness and possibly obesity.

Many lonely people remember their parents as having been critical of themselves or their friends in childhood. Families in which there is significant conflict, and marriages that end in divorce can induce children to experience anxiety about abandonment, feelings of rejection and guilt, and fears of being different from peers.

On the other hand, parents who model good attitudes and positive ways of relating to others, and who promote a good self-concept in their children, help their children to be successful in social interactions. The family functions as a source of interpersonal involvement, the context for the acquisition of interpersonal skills, and a secure base from which to establish peer relationships. When these are healthy, unnecessary loneliness can be prevented.

Overeating is sometimes the salve for loneliness, but the resulting weight problem only makes it more difficult for the lonely person to reach out and overcome that loneliness. Learning how to initiate and maintain social relationships is one element in overcoming loneliness. Using positive self-talk and avoiding self-criticism and thoughts focused on unworthiness are also important.

Action steps must be initiated as well. These include working around time and money constraints, and if necessary changing your immediate environment. Ultimately, it is important to develop aloneness skills. Whenever possible, steps should be taken to prevent loneliness.

Summary

Two other emotions that make weight management difficult are anger and loneliness. When anger is vented inappropriately, it can produce turmoil and stress that ultimately leads to overeating. Likewise, the person who has difficulty owning or expressing her anger often finds herself stuffing down her feelings with food.

Anger can be a healthy emotion; it tells you when your needs are not being met and action should be taken. On the other hand, anger that defeats your ability to get what you want out of life is unhealthy anger. It is important to be able to tell the difference, and to manage anger so that it serves you.

Loneliness can also be a source of unwanted eating. People who experience food as their best friend are basically lonely. In lieu of human connectedness, they fill up the emptiness with food and eating.

Meaningful relationships are essential for psychological health. Likewise, weight management success depends in part on overcoming loneliness.

References

1. Grieger, R. (1982). Anger problems. In R. Brieger and I. Z. Grieger (Eds.), *Cognition and Emotional Distrubance.* New York: Human Sciences Press (pp. 46–75).

2. Novaco, R. W. (1978). Anger and coping with stress: Cognitive-behavioral interventions. In J. P. Foreyt and D. P. Rathjen (Eds.), *Cognitive Behavior therapy: Research and Applications.* New York: Plenum Press (pp. 135–174).

3. McKay, M., Rogers, P. D. & McKay, J. (1989). *When Anger Hurts.* Oakland, CA: New Harbinger.

Chapter 9

Coping With Binge Eating

GINNY DESCRIBED what she called a binge that she had succumbed to in the past week:

"The candy was there, and at first I had just one little piece. Then I went back and got another and another until it was all gone. It tasted so good I didn't want to stop eating it. I told myself it had been a rough day and I deserved the treat, but afterwards I wished I hadn't done it."

Maureen told how binge eating made staying at goal weight impossible:

"Losing weight is easy for me, but once I get to my goal weight, I start binging, and I eventually regain all the weight I lost and more. I'm always thinking about food. When I'm dieting, I'm planning what I'll fix to eat and when I'll eat. When I get to goal weight, I think about all the foods I couldn't have before that I want to have now. I know I shouldn't but I go ahead and eat something I know is fattening, and then I feel bad. I'm afraid I'll regain weight again. I get so upset that I just keep eating. That's crazy. I don't know why I do it; I'm not even hungry. I think I'm addicted to food. I can't control myself. I feel guilty and I get down on myself for being so weak. I wish I had the willpower to stay on a diet."

Laura described her situation:

"When I get depressed, which is a lot of the time, I just get this overwhelming compulsion to eat. I'll eat just about anything, but I prefer sweets, junk foods, and fast foods—you know, candy, pastries, ice cream, chips, pretzels, corn curls, Big Macs, milk shakes—anything I can get my hands on easily. I won't eat when anyone's around, so no one really knows what I'm doing. Sometimes I overeat like this for days. Then I go on a diet to compensate. Sometimes I fast for several days. I can gain ten pounds in one week and lose it again just as fast. All the time I hate myself. I'm afraid I can't stop, and it scares me. I'm disgusted with myself. I'm worthless and don't deserve to eat at all."

All three of these women see themselves as binge eaters, but are they? Most people call any kind of unwanted, unplanned, or impulsive overeating a "binge," even if relatively few calories have been consumed. But occasional episodes of unwanted eating don't always constitute a binge. They may just be cases of simple overeating.

Just what constitutes overeating depends on your definition. Overeating may be eating past the point of satiety—past the point of feeling full. Overeating could be eating past some arbitrary limit, such as eating past some predetermined caloric level established by a diet. Or overeating may be eating in excess of the amount of calories required to maintain a stable weight, though just what this level is in any individual case may be difficult to determine.

Although all of these may be examples of "overeating," none of them is necessarily a binge. Binge eating is defined as eating an amount of food in a short period of time (usually within a two hour period) that is definitely larger than most people would eat during a similar period of time and feeling one can't stop eating or control what or how much one is eating.[1]

Binge eating—the kind that constitutes an eating disorder—has certain characteristics. Physical hunger is not usually what triggers binge eating. Eating may be much more rapid than usual, and the binge eater may eat until she feels uncomfortably full. Alternatively, the binger eater may eat more or less continuously throughout the day, with no planned mealtimes. Often the binge eater eats alone because she is embarrassed and doesn't want anyone to know how much she is eating.

A key feature of binge eating that has become an eating disorder is that the binge eater suffers considerable psychological distress. She feels disgusted with herself, depressed, or guilty after binge eating. Finally, to be categorized as an eating disorder, binge eating must occur at least twice a week for six months or more.

Simple Overeating

All binges are episodes of overeating, but not all overeating episodes qualify as binges. What Ginny experienced was simple overeating, even though in her mind she had binged. Eating the candy may have been undesirable behavior, but when such behavior happens only occasionally, and is accompanied by few or mild emotional reactions, it falls into the category of simple overeating.

Simple overeating rarely involves eating the large number of calories—sometimes 5,000 to 10,000 at one time—that a true eating binge usually involves. Sometimes simple overeating is a transient response to emotional stress, or it may be triggered by the situation—for example, food is available or there is social pressure to overeat.

Everyone—fat or thin—overeats now and then, and if asked why, they may simply refer to "liking the taste," and not wanting to stop. In contrast to the true binge eater, the person involved in simple overeating does not feel out of control the way a true binge eater does. The simple overeater chooses to eat inappropriately, usually by finding some rationale for the behavior.

Appropriate strategies for overcoming simple overeating are to exercise better control over the environment, to learn coping skills for dealing with social influences, and to avoid rationalizing that permits inappropriate behavior. Learning to improve thinking skills and to use coping self-talk is important for avoiding simple overeating. Overcoming serious binge eating requires additional tactics.

Binge Eating as a Disorder

Both Maureen and Laura felt they had little or no control over their binge eating. In Maureen's case, her loss of control and her binge eating alternated with fairly long periods of good control, and relative absence of binge eating behavior when she was dieting down to goal weight. Only when she reached goal weight did binge eating become a real problem.

Both Maureen and Laura felt guilt and shame as a result of their binging behavior, and both tend to be self-critical as a result. Laura, in particular, appears to be distressed by her binge eating.

As with all true binge eaters, Maureen and Laura's binge eating is preceded by anticipatory anxiety, and involves excessive eating of food which is usually gulped or eaten quickly. The eating takes place in private, and is carried to the point of satiation, producing feelings of guilt, shame, and self-condemnation.

Binge eating that involves episodic overeating, the loss of control, psychological distress, and certain characteristics such as rapid eating, eating without hunger, and eating in secret is a serious problem. When such binge eating is followed by vomiting or the use of laxatives to compensate for the overeating, it is termed "bulimia nervosa." Other ways to compensate for binge eating without purging include restrictive dieting, skipping meals, engaging in strenuous exercise, using diuretics, using amphetamines or diet pills, and chewing without swallowing and spitting out the food.

Bulimia nervosa, which involves binge eating and compensatory behavior to avoid weight gain, is most common among people of normal weight. However, recent research suggests that from 25% to 50% of obese people, mostly females, engage in binge eating without either vomiting or using laxatives to compensate.[2,3] Such people appear to be more severely obese and are more likely to relapse.[5] A new diagnosis for this group of "binge eating disorder" has been proposed for the fourth edition of the American Psychiatric Association's Diagnostic and Statistical Manual.[1]

People who have a binge eating disorder or who binge and purge have a characteristic way of thinking that seems to create and perpetuate their eating problem. They tend to be excessively perfectionistic, and demand of themselves superior achievement. They attempt to adhere rigidly to unrealistic goals, and the slightest deviation is condemned as a failure. They attribute any "failure" to their own inadequacies, and neglect to give adequate attention to external factors that play a role.

As a result of taking upon themselves all responsibility for outcomes, they feel generally inadequate, insecure, worthless, and out of control. This leads to the experience of discomfort in expressing emotions toward others, a sense of alienation from others, and a general reluctance to form close relationships.

Characteristics of Binge Eating

Prevalence

It was once widely believed that there was an "epidemic" of eating disorders on college campuses. The professional literature reported high rates of bulimia nervosa, and *Newsweek* magazine dubbed 1981 the "year of the binge-purge syndrome."

The problem in determining prevalence was that different researchers used different definitions and criteria to decide what constituted disordered eating. As a result, some studies included people who were simple overeaters, while others excluded all but the most severe binge eaters.

More recent and rigorous research has found that while simple overeating is quite common, bulimia nervosa is much less common than formerly believed—less than 3% in the general public, around 7% in weight control programs, and about 35% among Overeaters Anonymous members. People with a binge eating disorder—involving true binge eating but no compensatory behavior—were far more common, especially among people participating in weight control programs. About 30% of those joining weight control programs can be characterized as having a binge eating disorder. Among Overeaters Anonymous members, the proportion is closer to 70%.

However, the more important question may not to be how many people can be classified as bulimic or binge eaters, but rather what are the conditions that establish and maintain binge eating?

Description of a Binge

Binges may occur nearly constantly—from two or three times a week to five to ten times a day—or they may be more intermittent. They may last minutes, hours, or even days. Nearly 52% of the subjects in one study reported that the average length of a binge-eating episode for them was 15 minutes to one hour. Only 5% said a binge lasted more than four hours. Although any type of food may be consumed in a binge, the most preferred foods are described as sweets, junk foods, snack foods, and fast foods.

Binge eating shares many of the characteristics of a compulsion, which is "a behavior that a person has to do (not wants to do), because of some internal pressure (not external coercion), which makes little logical sense, and results in negative emotional consequences." The essence of a compulsion is its "push-pull" nature. The food beckons, while the binger tries to resist taking the first bite for fear of losing total control. There is an ambivalence toward food—a love/hate relationship.

Maureen's experience with binge eating, once she reached goal weight, was much like this. As long as food was the enemy and kept under control with dieting, she was safe. Once food became fair game, as it did when she reached goal weight, she no longer was safe. Maureen did not know how to treat food except as an enemy, to be hated and feared. Even eating moderately signaled no longer being in control, and binge eating followed.

Binge eating may also take on the complexion of an addiction. An addiction is characterized by the feeling that there is never enough. There is an insistent craving for food, and eating in moderation is not enough.

While a recovering alcoholic can handle his urges with complete abstinence, a binge eater obviously cannot abstain from food. For the binge eater, abstinence really means abstaining from food abuse and inappropriate snacking (but not necessarily all snacking, since planned, healthy snacks can be appropriate).

As with other kinds of addictions, binge eating produces certain consequences for the binger, and some of these serve to maintain the behavior. Stanton Peele, in his book, *How Much Is Too Much?: Healthy Habits or Destructive Addictions*, describes what an addiction can do:

1. *It eradicates awareness* . . . of what is hurting or troubling [her] . . .

2. *It hurts other involvements* . . . the person then turns increasingly toward the experience of [her] own source of gratification in life . . .

3. *It lowers self-esteem* . . .

4. *It is not pleasurable* . . . There is nothing pleasurable about the addiction cycle. . . what is "pleasurable" about addiction is the absence of feelings and thoughts that lead to pain. . .

5. *It is predictable* . . . [providing] a sureness of effect. (pp. 5-6)

Using Peele's description as a guide, P. A. Neuman and P. A. Halvorson, in their book, *Anorexia Nervosa and Bulimia: A Handbook for Counselors and Therapists*, describe how binge eating and the binge/purge cycle can take on the appearance of an addiction:

Binge eating and the binge/purge cycle temporarily ward off the pain, anxiety, and consciousness of the person's immediate problem. This is usually accomplished by triggering a whole sequence of events—food must first be obtained, a place to eat it must be located, and for some binge eaters a place to regurgitate must be found. The guilt and self-disgust that set in often lead to a repetition of the cycle. All of this functions to ward off the anxiety that is associated with the real problem. Binging becomes a strategy for avoidance.

To the extent that the binger becomes increasingly food-oriented or focused on her concerns about binge eating, other interests suffer, including close relationships, budgetary considerations, and health. Often the binger tries to keep her binge eating a secret from friends or a spouse by telling lies or otherwise covering up.

Her constant preoccupation with food or her weight can make it difficult even to carry on a conversation, and can further impede the relationship. The binge "habit" requires money, and overdrawn checking accounts and financial difficulties are not unusual. Health is likely to suffer in a variety of ways that will be discussed later in this chapter.

The binge eater views her behavior as weird or disgusting, which leads to guilt and self-hate. The more out of control she feels, the more her self-confidence and self-esteem sink. She may develop a negative and unhealthy (in the sense that it contributes to emotional upset) body image, which further exacerbates the binge eating.

While the binger certainly likes food, she does not generally take real pleasure in the food consumed during a binge. There is no active savoring of it. In fact, the food is eaten so rapidly that it is not even tasted. As one woman reported, "After the first bite or two, it could be cardboard and it wouldn't matter." Some binge eaters report that the food creates a "buzz," but it can take several days of nearly constant eating for this effect to be experienced.

The "pleasure" produced by the binge is not in the eating and tasting of the food, but in the avoidance of the feelings and thoughts from which the binge allows the binger to escape. (There may be some initial satisfaction of hunger as well, since many binges follow a period of fasting or dieting. In fact, getting too hungry as the result of fasting or restrictive dieting is a significant trap that can trigger another binge.)

Because the binge tends to occur in private, the usual social reasons for eating food are not present. There is no joy or celebration in the eating—only relief. Likewise, purging, if it is done, is not pleasurable either. But like the binge, it too serves a purpose that is reinforcing—it helps reduce anxiety about gaining weight and guilt related to the eating.

A binge is predictable. It works every time to block the real problem from consciousness, and to reduce the anxiety that goes with that problem. The binge provides structure and demands time, so that the binger does not have to deal with the confusion or time demands of the rest of her world.

Characteristics of the Binge Eater

Often the binge eater is a "good dieter." She may report a history of successful diets, where weight loss was achieved, but then not maintained.

In many cases, the binge eater fits the description of a *restrained eater*. She is constantly concerned about dieting, weight, and weight loss. She generally maintains strict control over eating; but certain circumstances, such as having a glass of wine or committing a small dietary indiscretion, can undo her control and trigger binging.

The effort required to restrain eating—to diet—may itself trigger binge eating. The dieter holds herself to very high dieting standards, and becomes upset when she violates her diet. She has a tendency to be inflexible and to overdo things. She may also abuse alcohol or drugs.

The essential problem with the restrained eater seems to be in the way she thinks about dieting, her weight, and herself. She usually holds herself to unrealistic dieting or weight standards. When she breaches these, she is likely to become self-critical, which produces guilt, anger directed at the self, binge eating, and a new cycle of perfectionistic and unrealistic dieting resolutions.

When guilt, self-criticism, and anger directed at the self are taken to the extreme, the binger may become a *self-hater*. Negative beliefs about the self, and persistent self-critical thoughts keep self-esteem low, and contribute to depression. The self-hater has an unhealthy body image—an overly negative perception that her body is not acceptable, unattractive, or even ugly, which produces painful emotions and often self-destructive behavior.

Some symptoms of an unhealthy body image include feeling ashamed to be seen in public, avoiding seeing one's self in mirrors or plate glass windows, or general embarrassment about one's body. The self-hater vents anger on herself, and overeating is a self-destructive behavior that serves in part as self-punishment.

The self-test, *How's Your Body Image?* (page 187), which has been used in research to identify bingers and those who have an unhealthy body image, is useful for assessing whether a poor body image is involved in triggering your binges

A binge eater may be a *people pleaser*. She may put other people's needs before her own. Her husband's needs, her children's needs, her parent's needs, the demands of the job, the demands of her organization all come first. She may not even be aware that she has left no time to meet her own needs. Her energies are directed outward to other people, and when it comes to herself, the well has often run dry. If she is aware of her own needs, she may not assert her right to have them met. Beliefs about her proper role, and how a "good mother" or "good wife" should act, keep her from acting on her own behalf.

Pleasing others goes very deep for many women; religious teachings sometimes place high value on personal sacrifice and define personal need as "selfishness" that is sinful. In the zest to reap the joy that comes with giving, and to avoid the sin of egoism, the lesson may be lost that the truly generous person is not herself desperately racked with unmet needs.

The person who does things ostensibly for others may really be looking for a hidden bargain—i.e., "If I'm nice and do this, I'll get that." But when all her sacrifice and self-denial doesn't pay off, the feelings of hurt and anger that result can trigger binge eating. She is not even aware that her manipulative and self-seeking actions, cloaked in the guise of selflessness, create her painful emotions, and cause her to attempt to cope with them—by binging. She may even become a vengeful binger.

The *vengeful binger* eats to punish someone else or to thwart another's desires. The vengeful binger perceives herself as having been wronged, slighted, or hurt in some way by another, and overeating takes on a flavor of "take that, you cur." One young woman continually binged and maintained her obesity as a reaction against her mother, who had always been thin and concerned about image and appearance, even though her mother lived 3000 miles away. Vengeful binging can be a means of trying to hurt others for real or imagined wrongs, or it can be an attempt to arouse feelings of guilt in others by setting it up so the binge is "their fault."

A binge eater may be someone who simply has developed bad eating and dieting habits. The *bad habits binger* is likely to skip meals, and to go without food for extended periods; meals and eating have a high level of variability.

She may indulge in extreme dieting, fad diets, and self-denial. She doesn't manage her environment well, and as a result, food that prompts a binge is easily available. Or she may eat an excessive amount of sugary or junk foods, which contribute to a physical state that makes her even more prone to binging.

Frequently the binger uses binge eating to escape from negative feelings or stressful situations. The *stressed binger* worries about things, is tense, and feels anxious. Binging provides a relief from these feelings. If there is an issue or problem she doesn't want to have to face, binging provides an alternative, and relieves the unpleasant feelings that come with thinking about the stressful situation. The stressed binger may come to believe she is a "food addict."

Some people who binge can't identify any cause for their binging. The *blocked binger* may be out of touch with her emotions, or may be suppressing an emotionally-charged issue with which she would rather not deal. A person who has been the victim of rape or childhood sexual abuse may have suppressed this memory, and may now be using food and binging to cope with flashbacks or resurgent emotions related to the memory. Or the blocked binger may be unconsciously avoiding having to face a present-day problem

Self-Test 9.1

How's Your Body Image?

	Never	Sometines	Often	Always
1. I dislike seeing myself in mirrors.	0	1	2	3
2. When I shop for clothing, I am more aware of my weight problem, and consequently I find shopping for clothes somewhat unpleasant.	0	1	2	3
3. I'm ashamed to be seen in public.	0	1	2	3
4. I prefer to avoid engaging in sports or public exercise because of my appearance.	0	1	2	3
5. I feel somewhat embarrassed about my body in the presence of someone of the opposite sex.	0	1	2	3
6. I think my body is ugly.	0	1	2	3
7. I feel that other people must think my body is unattractive.	0	1	2	3
8. I feel that my family or friends may be embarrassed to be seen with me.	0	1	2	3

Source: J.D. Nash and L.H. Ormiston, *Taking Charge of Your Weight and Well-Being*, Bull Publishing Company, Palo Alto, CA, 1978. Used with permission. Also known as the *Negative Self-Image Scale* and the *Jackson Body Image Scale*, this instrument has been used extensively in research on binge eating. See R.C. Hawkins, II and P.E. Clement, "Binge Eating: Measurement Problem and a Conceptual Model," in R.C. Hawkins, II, W.J. Fremouw and P.E. Clement, *The Binge-Purge Syndrome*, Springer Publishing Company, New York, NY, 1984. Also see S. Popkess (1981). "Assessment scales for determining the cognitive-behavior repertoire of the obese subject," *Western Journal of Nursing Research, 3,* 199.

that appears to have no good resolution, such as the dilemma between continuing to put up with sexual harassment or confronting the boss to try and stop the harassment.

A binger feels more or less out of control in the face of food. At the same time she fears fatness. The binger's reaction to a binge is further emotional upset and self-deprecating thoughts.

The real problem with a binge is not the overeating itself, but the meaning the binger gives to the overeating. She takes the binge as evidence that she can't cope, that she is helpless, and that she is worthless. While the

Self-Test 9.1

How's Your Body Image? (continued)

	Never	Sometines	Often	Always
9. I find myself comparing myself with other people to see if they are heavier than I am.	0	1	2	3
10. I find it difficult to enjoy activities because I am self-conscious about my physical appearance.	0	1	2	3
11. Feeling guilty about my weight problem preoccupies most of my thinking.	0	1	2	3
12. My thoughts about my body and physical appearance are negative and self-critical.	0	1	2	3

Now, add up the number of points
you have circled in each column: ___ + ___ + ___ = ___

Score Interpretation

The lowest possible score is "0," and this indicates a positive body image. The highest possible score is "36," and this indicates an unhealthy body image. A score higher than "14" suggests a tendency toward an unhealthy body image.

If you have a score higher than "14," you need to challenge the negative beliefs you hold about yourself and change your self-talk to make it less self-critical. Review Chapter 3, which discussed how to "think smart," and Chapter 4 on self-talk, for details on how to do this.

more moderate bingers may display only a few of these characteristics, more serious bingers show many of them.

Moderate vs. Serious Bingers

Bingers vary in the severity of their affliction. In a study designed to differentiate between less serious and more serious binges, researchers found that 55% of their subjects were *moderate bingers*.[6] These people tended to react to a dietary slip-up by eating even more.

Even though they binged, however, they tended to be more tolerant of their lapse in self-control than the other bingers. They reported less guilt and self-hate. Although they experienced intense food cravings, and were also somewhat preoccupied with food and eating, they felt these symptoms less intensely than did the more serious bingers. Much like Maureen, whose story was told at the beginning of this chapter, the moderate binger may experience episodic periods of poor control, interspersed with periods of good control.

In contrast to moderate bingers, *serious bingers*, which constituted 23% of the subjects in the study, felt a more pervasive lack of control over their eating urges, and experienced an almost constant preoccupation with eating or not eating. Their overeating tended to be much more extreme than that of the moderate bingers, and their fear of losing control was so intense that they often reported being unable to keep food in their homes. Serious bingers ate greater amounts of food, experienced more guilt and self-hate after the binge, and used more extreme dieting methods.

Serious bingers also tended to have other problems that made their binging worse, including depression and less ability to deal with life problems. They tended to be under-assertive and to display extreme deference to authority figures. In addition, serious bingers tend to have difficulty dealing effectively with others, be ambivalent about sex or have unsatisfying sexual involvements, hold a negative self-image, be overly dependent on others, have conflicts about achievement, feel insecure, or show uncertainty about their identity.

The other 22% of the people in this study also reported significant overeating, but none of the conflict and self-hate that is so characteristic of the binge syndrome. The researchers called this person an *indulger*. These people overeat because they enjoy eating. They don't feel out of control and they reported little negative emotional response to their overeating. While the binger struggles with the urge to eat, the indulger approaches eating without ambivalence.

Dieting is extremely difficult for the indulger because she likes food so much, whereas dieting is something the binger generally does quite well, at least part of the time. Because they eat a lot of food, indulgers may appear to be bingers. In fact, their's is a different kind of eating disorder.

Other Types of Eating Disorders

For some time bulimia was believed to be a subset of another eating disorder, anorexia nervosa. In fact, anorexia nervosa is a complex emotional disorder that launches its victims on a course of frenzied dieting in pursuit of excessive thinness. Some people afflicted with anorexia nervosa literally starve themselves to death. Although some anorexics may display binge eating behavior, bulimia is now distinguished as an eating disorder quite separate from anorexia nervosa.

Long-Term Effects of Binging and Purging

Serious binging and purging behavior takes a heavy toll. In addition to the psychological problems of depression, low self-esteem, and unhealthy body image, which can even lead to suicide, there are serious physical side effects.

Binging overloads the stomach, and can cause it to rupture. Binging on sugary foods sends blood sugar sky rocketing, causing huge amounts of insulin to be released in response. This alone may cause a precipitous drop in blood sugar level, triggering symptoms of hypoglycemia—shaking, irritability, inability to concentrate. If vomiting is used to purge the sugary food, this, too, can cause a dive in blood sugar (due to an insulin dump reaction).

Purging has other serious side effects, which can produce medical complications. Frequent vomiting may cause tears in the esophagus, and the acid in the vomit can rot the teeth, irritate the throat, and cause the salivary glands to swell. Abuse of laxatives and/or diuretics can cause the bowels to lose tone and become less able to function on their own. Dry skin, facial puffiness, bloodshot eyes, chronic indigestion, urinary infections, irregular menstrual periods, and impaired kidney function are all common consequences. Perhaps most serious of all are the fluid and electrolyte abnormalities, which can precipitate fatal heart problems.

For these reasons, it is recommended that serious bingers who also purge get medical and well as psychiatric treatment. In addition to providing appropriate treatment for bulimia-related medical problems, obtaining an initial medical work-up may help to rule out hypoglycemia and a possible neurological basis for the binging behavior.

Symptoms of Neurological Binge Eating

In a small minority of cases, binge eating may be caused by a problem in the brain, possibly in the appetitive centers of the hypothalamus. Symptoms that may indicate the existence of a neurologically-based disorder of impulse control include:

1.   *Unusual sensation or aura prior to a binge.* Just prior to indulging in a binge, the neurogenic binge eater may experience an unusual physical sensation or aura—such as flashes of light or unusual smells. The binger may report having a very poor memory of the episode, but be able to recall feeling a sense of "strangeness" just prior to the binge.

2.   *Ego-alien experience of the binge.* Some neurogenic binge eaters feel that their true self is not involved in the binge eating, that something or someone outside themselves is involved with the binge.

3.   *No good psychological explanation.* Usually there is no psychological

pattern (e.g., serious depression, stress reactions, etc.) that can be associated with the binge eating.

4. *Unusual post-binge symptoms.* Most bingers report feeling full and falling asleep after a binge, or feeling a relief from tension, but a few neurogenic bingers report other symptoms that psychogenic bingers do not report. These include extended periods of sleep or loss of consciousness, confusion, memory loss or disruption, headaches, or loss of bladder control on or after awakening.

What Can Be Done?

In the case of a neurologically-determined binger, the first step is to consult a professional and obtain an EEG. If it shows an abnormal pattern, medication has been shown to produce improvement in 70% of patients.

On the other hand, if the EEG is normal, this does not rule out a neurological basis to the binging problem. Indeed, there is a 40% to 50% probability that the test will be read as showing normal when in fact it is abnormal. Trying prescribed medication may still be appropriate. With or without medication, attention needs to be given to the psychosocial factors involved in binge eating.

Self-Esteem and Binge Eating

Some experts suggest that binging behavior is related to socially-induced evaluations related to self-esteem. That is, women in American society are led to believe that their self-worth and value are dependent upon their body and their appearance. Critical self-evaluations lead to a negative self-image, and possibly an unhealthy body image for many women. Indeed, the national obsession with slimness and calorie counting affects women, for the most part, and not men.

Men learn to evaluate a woman, at least initially, on the basis of her body and her appearance. This, it is contended, produces anger and resentment on the part of women, which leads to binging behavior. However, while this may explain binging behavior for women, men binge too, and it does not address their problem.

Whether or not a negative self-image and associated emotions come primarily from values imposed by society, certain ways of thinking are at the heart of virtually all binge eating. A binger may have the "dieter's mentality" of the restrained eater, or she may distort and deny information available to her. Four kinds of thought patterns may trigger or exacerbate binge eating:

1. A tendency to attribute the cause of inappropriate eating behavior to the self rather than the situation or external factors, which results in self-blame;

2. perfectionistic, either/or thinking, which leads to setting unrealistic goals and holding oneself to excessively high standards;

3. a failure to set priorities, leading among other things to putting others' needs first; and

4. magical thinking—looking for the easy or quick answer to a problem, rather than identifying the real problem and systematically dealing appropriately with it.

Certain ways of thinking not only make binge eating more likely, they lead to unpleasant emotions. The binger then attempts to deal with emotional arousal by using whatever means she has. Eating is one way (as is abusing alcohol or drugs, or compulsive gambling, or lighting up a cigarette). The ritual and effort involved in a binge is particularly effective for blotting out emotional arousal from another problem.

When a binger is suffering tension from some unresolved issue, and especially if she does not see how to resolve the issue, the binge provides a diversion and a relief. Binging relieves stressful feelings that come from having to cope with a change in routine or with something new. If the binger is bored, the binge gives her something to do. Anxiety associated with uncertainty about one's identity, and conflicts about achievement may prompt binging.

Under-assertiveness or extreme deference to authority figures may be at the base of some binging problems. Those who are shy or feel anxious in social situations may turn to binging to relieve their loneliness, or to deal with the anxiety they feel. The stressful feelings associated with coming into conflict with others, or having to confront something unpleasant can lead to avoidance and withdrawal, and can trigger an eating binge.

Sometimes, the binger has blocked from awareness the source of the emotional upset. She may experience a "hunger" that is not satisfied. Her eating behavior is experienced as "prowling"—searching for something satisfying to eat, eating, but not feeling satisfied. In other cases, the binge may be used to keep out of consciousness a noxious situation or to keep blocked from awareness the memory of a painful event.

Overcoming Binge Eating

Begin With Assessment

Before you can make much progress in overcoming binge eating, you need to identify what seems to be triggering your eating binges. It is helpful to keep a record of binging behavior—what was eaten, the cues or circumstances that seemed to trigger the eating binge, the thoughts that went through your mind before, during, and after the binge, and the emotions or feelings that were involved. Also record what you did in reaction to the binge—vomit, fast, diet, exercise, and so forth.

Make copies of and use the *Binging Behavior Record* on page 195 to help you track and identify the particular circumstances involved in your binging. That is, what thoughts, feelings, and circumstances lead up to the binge, how do you experience the binge, and what do you do afterwards? Keep a record of these aspects of your binge behavior as long as necessary to get the information on your pattern. Usually this will require keeping track for several weeks. With this information, you will be better able to plan how to cope with binge eating.

Uncover Your Triggers

Another means of gaining a better understanding of what triggers your binging behavior is to complete the following self-test, *What Triggers Your Binges?* Your answers will suggest some of the things that lead up to binge eating for you.

Interpreting Your Assessment

Review the items you have checked in this self-test. Items are grouped by category— Social, Cognitive (thinking skills), Emotional, and Environmental. (Note that some items under one category might legitimately fit into another category. Thus, "can't sleep" fits under Environmental if you can't sleep because late eating or drinking alcohol before bed makes you wake up in the night. On the other hand, "can't sleep" would fit more appropriately under Emotional if it is associated with depression.)

Pay particular attention to the items you have rated "almost always" or "frequently." These are the ones that are most likely to trigger binge eating for you. Now note how you have rank ordered these items. If your number one item is in the Social category, this indicates you need to acquire more effective social skills related to that item. That is, you may need to learn how to communicate more effectively, or to handle conflict better, or to be more assertive, and so forth.

Likewise, the items you have checked in the Cognition category indicate you need to focus on improving your thinking skills. If so, review Chapter 3, on *Learning to "Think Smart."*

If you have rated any items in the Emotional category, you may need to learn how to handle emotional arousal better, or you may need to deal more effectively with the problems that are generating the emotional arousal. In this case, review Chapter 7, *Overcoming Depression and Anxiety*, and Chapter 8, *Managing Anger and Loneliness.*

If you have items in the Environmental category, you need to work on

Self-Test 9.2

What Triggers Your Binges?

What things seem to trigger a binge for you? Check all that apply and then rate those you have checked, to indicate how frequently the items you have checked trigger binge eating for you. After you have finished rating each of the items you have checked, go back over these and rank order each of the items you rate "Almost Always" or "Frequently," giving a "1" to the item that is most often a problem for you, a "2" for the next most frequent problem, and so forth, until you have rank ordered all such items.

Rank Order	Almost Always	Frequently	Sometimes	Rarely
Social				
_____ trying to please others	____	____	____	____
_____ conflict with someone	____	____	____	____
_____ having to deal with certain people	____	____	____	____
_____ being teased or put down by someone	____	____	____	____
Cognitive				
_____ not meeting the standards I set for myself	____	____	____	____
_____ worrying or feeling bad about my weight	____	____	____	____
_____ thoughts about sexual relations	____	____	____	____
_____ having to cope with a change in my routine or with something new	____	____	____	____
_____ needing to resolve something or make a decision	____	____	____	____
_____ trying to avoid eating a particular food	____	____	____	____
_____ breaking my diet	____	____	____	____
_____ craving a particular food (e.g., chocolate)	____	____	____	____
_____ thoughts about how unattractive my body is	____	____	____	____
_____ worry about what others might think about me	____	____	____	____

(continued)

Self-Test 9.2

What Triggers Your Binges? (continued)

Rank Order	Almost Always	Frequently	Sometimes	Rarely
Cognitive (continued)				
_____ concerns that I don't measure up, or thoughts about how I've failed	_____	_____	_____	_____
_____ fear that my career success might slip away	_____	_____	_____	_____
_____ concerns about who I am in life	_____	_____	_____	_____
_____ concerns about my security	_____	_____	_____	_____
Emotional				
_____ feeling unhappy, sad or depressed	_____	_____	_____	_____
_____ feeling anxious or tense	_____	_____	_____	_____
_____ feeling angry or upset	_____	_____	_____	_____
_____ wanting something but I don't know what	_____	_____	_____	_____
_____ feeling there is never enough	_____	_____	_____	_____
_____ being bored or having time on my hands	_____	_____	_____	_____
_____ can't say; doesn't really seem to be connected to anything	_____	_____	_____	_____
Environmental				
_____ dieting	_____	_____	_____	_____
_____ feeling tired or fatigued	_____	_____	_____	_____
_____ hungry	_____	_____	_____	_____
_____ can't sleep	_____	_____	_____	_____
Other				
_____ other (please specify)	_____	_____	_____	_____
_____	_____	_____	_____	_____
_____	_____	_____	_____	_____
_____	_____	_____	_____	_____

Binging Behavior Record

Time /Day of Week	Food Eaten	What Made You Binge? Cues?	Thoughts & Emotions Before	Thoughts & Emotions During	Thoughts & Emotions After	What Did You Do After The Binge?

your behavior patterns and habits, and perhaps change some ways of doing things.

Compare your results on this self-test with the records you kept of your binging behavior to help you assess where you need to focus your efforts.

Immediate Steps You Can Take to Cope Better

1. *Focus on stabilizing weight.* When binging behavior is a serious problem, it needs to be attended to first, and the focus should be on stabilizing weight, not trying to lose weight. Avoid restrictive dieting until the binging is under control.

2. *Evaluate the effect of sugar on your binging.* Many binge eaters binge on sweets. One study concluded that the intake of sugary foods increased the probability of binging. Subjects in this study were more likely to engage in a binge, or to binge for a longer period of time if sweet foods were involved.

There has been some speculation that binging may be associated with episodic hypoglycemia, and this argues for eliminating sugar from the diet in an attempt to prevent this possibility. Some people believe themselves to be "sugarholics," and go so far as to hold that sugar (and other refined carbohydrates) are to the binger what alcohol is to the alcoholic. They maintain that it is frustrating and self-defeating to try to eat sweets in small amounts, and advocate abstinence as the best policy.

Although there may be some people for whom total abstinence from sugar is easier in the long run, a better approach for most people is to learn to eat occasional sweets. For many people, making a food off-limits creates a "forbidden fruit" effect, and can itself trigger binging. Rather, a phased approach to learning to live with sweets may be in order.

If you find that your binging (as well as your other eating) involves a lot of sugar or sugary foods, begin by *temporarily* eliminating all sugar from your diet. Eliminate not only foods that are obviously high in sugar, but seek to eliminate those with hidden sugar—e.g., some cereals, soft drinks, and certain processed foods. Abstain from eating sugar for a week or two, and observe how your behavior, as well as your mood, is affected. You are likely to discover you have more energy and feel less depressed.

Then gradually allow yourself to add sugar back to your diet. Continue to avoid, as much as possible, sources of hidden sugar, but allow yourself a sugary treat now and then, if you wish.

Be sure to manage your self-talk at all times. Tell yourself that you don't need or really want to eat sugar, that you don't like anything that tastes too sweet. Tell yourself that you are in charge and in control of sugar, that you are not "addicted" in any way, that you can handle it. If you find yourself thinking that you can't resist or that you crave sweets, use thought stopping and reassert that you are in charge.

If, after a fair trial, you find you still can't handle sugar, you should consider refraining from it altogether. Keep in mind that the "forbidden fruit" effect comes about because of the way you choose to look at the situation; you can make abstinence easier by the way you think about it and by the way you talk to yourself.

3. *Manage the environment.* When you are first trying to get in control of binging, it is important to manage the environment carefully to ensure that it does not make binging more likely.

Eliminate cues to eat. Don't have problem food in the house. Plan and manage your time so that there is no unstructured time. Plan to be out of the house if possible, and get involved in engaging activities. To avoid getting overly hungry, don't skip meals. Whenever possible, arrange to eat with other people.

Once you feel more in control and the incidence of binging has been reduced significantly, you can begin to relax your prohibitions. Although it is wise to keep your environment fairly free of cues to eat, it is also important to learn to live with food and opportunities to eat. Rigid control over the environment will not work over the long-term, but it can be helpful in the short-term in getting back your sense of balance.

4. *Set up choices.* Feeling out of control is the hallmark of binge eating. You can begin to regain the experience of being in control by setting up choices.

First, before the eating that might be the start of a binge, ask yourself, "What do I really want?" Is it the food you are about to eat, or is it relief from tension or something else? If you are hungry, go ahead and eat, reminding yourself that you are making a conscious choice to do so.

But if it is really something else you want, take other appropriate action. If you are feeling tense, do a relaxation exercise or go for a walk. If you are feeling angry, allow yourself to express it appropriately, even if it means going outside and yelling at the top of your lungs.

If you feel you are about to binge, use imagery and do a mental "run through" beforehand. In your mind see yourself eating as you might imagine you are about to, and notice whether you are enjoying the food. Continue in your imagination to the end of the eating episode, including imagining yourself having the guilt and negative feelings that come after a binge.

If after this you decide not to binge, congratulate yourself and quickly turn your efforts to doing something enjoyable or productive—take a bubble bath or clean your closets, write a poem or paint a picture, visit an art gallery, or just write in your journal about this experience.

If you are about to binge, make a decision to do so. In a notebook you keep for this purpose, write down that you have decided to binge. Write down what you will eat, how much you will eat, and where you will eat. Try to choose a place where people are, such as a restaurant.

Once you have decided to binge, wait 15 minutes before actually starting the binge. After 15 minutes, go ahead and binge, but do it in a particular way: Give yourself permission to eat without guilt. Eat slowly and savor each bite.

Also leave yourself the option to decide not to binge. If you decide not to, write this decision down as well. Then be prepared to do something nice for yourself. Have a list ready of things you could do for yourself, so you can refer to it if necessary.

It may be difficult at first to set up choices as suggested here. You will probably have to try several times before succeeding in interrupting a binge by giving yourself a choice. Don't give up, however. If you pause for 15 minutes and then still binge, congratulate yourself for having paused, and commit yourself to trying again next time. Pat yourself on the back for whatever steps you took, regardless of whether they worked this time, and determine to try again when necessary.

Long-Term Steps for Coping With Binge Eating

1.   *Develop skills for creating a more positive lifestyle and for coping better with life problems.* Learn to be assertive. Withdrawing and avoiding doesn't solve things; it only creates more problems. Learn to communicate in such a way that you get your needs met. Learn how to say "no." Work towards overcoming passivity, dependency on others, and the need to unduly accommodate others. Learn how to give and take criticism and negative feedback.

Learn to live in the present. Many binge eaters live in the past or the future. When you are feeling emotional, ask yourself, "What tense am I in?" Bring your focus back to now.

2.   *Learn how to cope more effectively with emotions.* Talk out feelings, rather than stuffing them down. Learn to label emotions correctly—e.g., don't confuse anxiety with hunger. Learn how to tolerate some anxiety, or how to reduce physical arousal through relaxation, meditation, imagery, or exercise. Learn to delay the impulse to eat. Learn to express emotion appropriately. Review Chapter 7, *Managing Painful Emotions.*

3.   *Learn to "think smart."* Develop a greater awareness of thinking traps such as perfectionism, applying rigid rules, labeling, and magical thinking, and learn to avoid them. Challenge negative beliefs you hold about yourself and develop "self-soothing skills." Evaluate and set your priorities in order to

make a reasonable commitment. Avoid using "toxic" words, such as can't, never, forever, always. Review Chapter 3, *Learning to "Think Smart."*

4.   *Become more tolerant.* Be more tolerant of your slips. Learn to recover sooner, before a small slip becomes a major setback. Build in little treats, and never make some food illegal or off limits. Making certain foods taboo focuses your energy on being vigilant not to eat the illegal food, and forces the desire for that food into consciousness. The energy devoted to being vigilant against an infraction creates tension that can actually increase the likelihood of having a setback.

Most of all, give yourself time to recover. Overcoming binge eating isn't accomplished in a day. It will take many tries and many small setbacks before you gain confidence in your ability to prevent or overcome a binge. Even then, occasional eating indiscretions are likely. After all, everyone overeats now and then. It's really a matter of who's in charge—you, or the food.

5.   *Undertake and maintain regular, moderate exercise.* Exercise not only stimulates the metabolism to speed up, and reduces body fat, it causes the body to produce substances in the brain that are associated with feelings of calmness and relaxation. To the degree that binging is triggered by stress and upset, exercise is a potent remedy. Be careful not to overdo or become perfectionistic about your exercise. Keep it fun!

Summary

Overeating and binging are not the same. In this chapter you learned the differences between what constitutes simple over-eating, binge eating, and bulimia.

One central factor in binge eating is a poor body image, and you were able to assess the degree to which you hold a negative body image. You also had the opportunity to assess what factors may be involved in causing you to binge. Finally, you learned what specific steps you can take now to cope with binge eating, as well as the long-term steps that will assure success in overcoming binge eating permanently.

References

1.   Spitzer, R.L., Devlin, M., Walsh, B.T., et al. (In press) Binge eating disorder: A multisite filed trial of the diagnostic criteria. *DSM-IV Casebook.* Washington, DC: American Psychiatric Press.

2.   Loro, A.D., & Orleans, C.S. (1981). Binge eating in obesity: Preliminary findings and guidelines. *Addictive Behaviors, 6,* 155–166.

3.   Marcus, M.D., Wing, R.R., & Lamparski, D.M. (1985). Binge eating and dietary restraint in obese patients. *Addictive Behaviors, 10,* 163–168.

4.   Telch, C.F., Agras, W.S., Rossiter, E.M., Wilfley, D., & Kenardy, J. (1990). Group cognitive-behavioral treatment for the nonpurging bulimic: An initial evaluation. *Journal of Consulting and Clinical Psychology, 58,* 629–635.

5.   Marcus, M.D., Wing, R.R., & Hopkins, J. (1988). Obese binge eaters: Affect, cognitions, and response to behavioral weight control. *Journal of Consulting and Clinical Psychology, 3,* 433–439.

6.   Gormally, J., Black, S., Daston, S., & Rardin, D. (1982). The assessment of binge eating severity among obese persons. *Addictive Behaviors, 7,* 47–55.

Chapter 10

Overcoming B­acksliding

HELEN DIETED ten months to get to goal weight, only to start gaining it all right back.

Susan joined the local YMCA fitness class, and for four months went faithfully three times a week. Then she caught a cold, and missed a couple of classes—she never went back.

Mary Ann was doing well controlling her eating. She hadn't had an eating binge in almost six weeks. Then one day she was going through her pantry and discovered a forgotten box of candy. She not only ate the entire box, she lost all control over her eating and gave up trying to manage her weight.

Wilma joined a weight control program and was doing well, having lost 19 pounds by the tenth week. Then her husband hurt his back. With the demands of her job, her young daughter, and now her incapacitated husband, Wilma decided she couldn't make time for her weight program. She dropped out.

Helen, Susan, Mary Ann, and Wilma all fell victim to backsliding.

Backsliding involves making a behavior change that results in at least partial success in achieving some desired goal—and then an erosion of commitment, and sometimes precipitous return to former habits. It means relinquishing control and losing whatever progress was made.

Usually backsliding starts with a single lapse—just one miss, one instance of "giving in to temptation," which escalates quickly to a full-blown relapse—a total collapse of resolve and commitment to change. Backsliding feels like making one step forward and two steps backward.

Psychologists have only recently begun to study the phenomenon of backsliding, which they call "relapse" or "recidivism."[1] By and large, this

---

A special debt of thanks is owed to G. Alan Marlatt, Ph.D., Director of Addictive Behaviors Research Center, and his colleagues at the University of Washington, for their work on relapse prevention, which forms the basis for much of this chapter.

research is done on clinical populations—people who join university sponsored programs for weight reduction. This research indicates that 90% to 95% of the people who succeed in losing weight in these programs eventually relapse—regain some or all of the weight lost. Losing weight is one thing; keeping it off is another.

Similarly, the data on exercise programs show that as much as three-quarters of those who start an exercise program eventually drop out—another way to backslide. Getting started with exercise may be an accomplishment in itself, but it does not necessarily lead to exercise becoming a permanent part of lifestyle.

In fact, the prospects for maintaining any significant change in lifestyle, whether involving diet, exercise, smoking, alcohol, or any other substantial change, are quite dismal. According to most research, backsliding is the likely result of most attempts to change a behavior pattern.

Backsliding is a significant problem. Understanding what causes backsliding, and learning how to overcome it can be crucial to your chances for lifelong success in maintaining new, healthier behaviors.

The Profile of Backsliding

Two-thirds of all backsliding occurs within the first ninety days after altering your behavior. It is usually triggered by a particular event or situation. Whether or not you are prepared to cope, and how you mentally react to a "triggering" situation, can determine whether or not you will backslide.

One of the biggest hazards is the first slip—having "just one," or "breaking the rules" just a little bit. As a result of the first slip, you are likely both to feel guilty, and to try and rationalize that backsliding is okay, or inevitable.

Not knowing how to recover from a small lapse—a first slip—virtually guarantees backsliding. Deciding that a first slip is terrible, or that you are bad or incapable of succeeding because you broke the rules just a little bit, moves you closer to full-blown backsliding—giving up all further efforts to change.

Backsliding, and the small lapses that lead to full-scale backsliding, often produces emotional upset and lowered self-esteem. Just how upset you get depends on several things.

If you feel the backsliding wasn't your fault, or you really didn't try too hard, you are likely not to feel so bad. On the other hand, the more effort you put into changing, or the more committed you are to the goal, the more upsetting backsliding is likely to be.

Backsliding after having maintained the new behavior pattern for a long time can be very upsetting. On the other hand, if you rationalize that "I wasn't able to keep up the new behavior patterns long enough for them to become habit," or "I knew all along I wouldn't be able to keep it off," backsliding is less likely to devastate you.

If someone you care about is angry or disapproving because you backslid, you are more likely to be upset. Backsliding by going out-of-control produces more negative emotions than backsliding as a result of a voluntary decision on your part to just quit trying. The more important the thwarted goal is to you, the more you will feel upset by backsliding.

Backsliding affects not only how you feel but how you think. It causes you to try and rationalize the actions that led to backsliding, so that you can stop feeling guilty about violating your commitment to change.

To find a good excuse, you may distort or deny the facts. Or you may unreasonably blame yourself totally for the backsliding, and as a result your self-esteem declines and your self-image suffers. Your self-confidence in your ability to cope takes a nose dive, and you develop an expectation for future failure.

Alternatively, if you unjustly blame someone else for the backsliding, you may create problems in your relationship with that person. If you place all the blame on the situation, failing to acknowledge your own accountability, you are less likely to learn from the experience, and to avoid future backsliding.

In order to justify having committed a small infraction, you may continue some "prohibited" behavior, thus impelling yourself from a single slip to full-blown backsliding. Or you may see the infraction as evidence of your inability to succeed, and decide to quit trying.

If, on the other hand, you are willing to view deviations from your commitment as opportunities from which to learn how to be more in charge of your behavior, you open the way to renewed commitment.

To see how slips can be valuable in your change efforts, you need to better understand the things that can cause backsliding, and what steps you can take to cope more effectively. Many things can contribute to backsliding, including high risk situations, errors in thinking, an unsupportive context, lack of coping skills, and an unbalanced lifestyle.

Dealing With High Risk Situations

When Susan got sick with a cold, and when Mary Ann discovered the forgotten box of candy in her pantry, they both unwittingly encountered a "high risk" situation. G. Alan Marlatt, the psychologist who first proposed the notion of a "high risk situation," broadly defines it as "any situation that poses a threat to the individual's sense of control and increases the risk of potential relapse." From his work, he has identified two general groups of high risk situations—Intrapersonal/environmental determinants and Interpersonal determinants.

1. *Intrapersonal/Environmental Determinants*

    Negative Emotions, Moods, or Feelings—Including experiencing frustration, anger, fear, anxiety, tension, depression, loneliness, sadness, boredom, worry, apprehension, grief, or loss, as well as stressful feelings related to such situations as examinations, promotions, public speaking, employment and financial difficulties, or personal misfortune or accident.

    Negative Physical States—Including experiencing unpleasant or painful physical or psychological experiences, such as pain, illness, injury, fatigue, having reactions associated with drugs or with withdrawal from an addictive substance, or reacting to hormonal or chemical imbalances such as those associated with diabetes, hyperglycemia, or Premenstrual Syndrome (PMS).

    Private Positive Emotions—Including desires for or actions intended to produce feelings of "getting high," pleasure, relaxation, or being secure, loved, accepted, or nurtured.

    Tests of Personal Control—Including thoughts that rationalize actions on the basis of having "just one," thoughts focusing on testing willpower, or overconfidence in one's capacity for moderate use.

    Urges or Temptations—Including responses to both sudden inclinations and to enduring desires to return to old habits.

2. *Interpersonal Determinants*

    Interpersonal Conflict Situations—Including relationships such as marriage, friendship, family interactions, and employer/employee relations, which involve frustration, anger, arguments, disagreements, fights, jealousy, discord, hassles, anxiety, fear, tension, apprehension, or guilt, or any interpersonal situation that involves any of these emotions.

    Social Influences—Including situations in which either an individual or a group actively uses pressure, coerces, tempts, coaxes, prepares, or makes a gift that influences another to return to old habits, or situations when such a return to old habits is prompted merely by observation of an individual or group engaging in the prohibited behaviors.

    Interpersonal Positive Emotions—Including social situations that generate feelings of pleasure, celebration, sexual excitement, freedom, and the like.

According to Marlatt, nearly 75% of all backsliding is triggered by three of these determinants—negative emotions, interpersonal conflict, and social influences.

Crisis Situations

Similarly, other research has identified three clusters of typical crisis situations for weight control.[2] Social mealtime situations, usually involving friends or family and taking place in a restaurant, were the most common. Spirits are often high, and negative emotions tend to be absent at these times.

A second cluster of crisis situations consisted of situations involving some kind of emotional upset, especially anger, but also including situations in which anxiety or depressed mood was associated. Most of these occurred when the dieter was alone, although sometimes others were present.

The third cluster, termed "low arousal," was characterized by eating while alone. The dieters reported feeling no particular emotions at such a time, though occasionally they felt tired or bored. These crisis situations seemed to involve relaxing, waiting, or being between other activities. Often food was present or easily available, or the dieter reported feeling hungry.

In order to substantially reduce the risk of backsliding, therefore, it is important to learn to cope with high risk or crisis situations that can prompt overeating. Skills are needed for coping with emotions, dealing more effectively with interpersonal conflict, and managing social influences and situations.

It is especially crucial to bring these skills to bear during the critical period—the first ninety days of a new behavior pattern. It is also important to know how to recover from a small lapse and not let one slip trigger full-blown backsliding.

How Backsliding Happens

Backsliding usually starts with a high risk or crisis situation. Most people don't recognize when they are in a high risk situation or how this can trigger backsliding. Helen couldn't understand why she periodically had the urge to bake things like pie, cake, or cookies, which she would then eat, despite the fact that she was making good progress in managing her weight. She knew these small lapses could eventually lead to total backsliding, as had happened in the past. By carefully analyzing the events that preceded the urge to bake, the reason became obvious.

She discovered that on the occasions when her husband was in a bad mood and refused to communicate with her, she got anxious and upset. To relieve these feelings and to get her mind off them, she would cook. A high risk situation for Helen was having her husband in a bad mood. Once she learned to identify this, she was able to plan more effective ways to cope, which put her on the road to overcoming backsliding.

Some high risk situations are more insidious. Jane had joined several weight reduction programs, and had lost 25 or 30 pounds each time. But she always dropped out of the program before reaching goal weight and quit trying to lose more or even to maintain the lower weight.

The high risk situation that led to Jane's backsliding was "creeping boredom." At the beginning of each program she felt very enthusiastic about losing weight and was excited about making the commitment to do so. Her thoughts focused on how good she would feel about herself when she could wear a skimpy bathing suit and how pleased her husband would be. She would anticipate the compliments everyone would give her and how much better she would feel by doing regular exercise.

Jane would start out each time really well, losing two to three pounds a week. By about the twelfth week, however, her enthusiasm would begin to wane. Counting calories became boring. Exercising became boring. Sure, she was getting compliments, and her husband was urging her not to give up this time, but the constant attention to dieting and exercising was getting to be a drag. Instead of thinking motivating thoughts, Jane would dwell on how slow and boring it all was.

The crisis situation for Jane involved boredom and having to tolerate the slow progress of weight loss. Her thinking gradually evolved from focusing on the benefits of losing weight and the costs of being fat to the costs of losing weight and the benefits of not trying. She would tell herself that eating "diet" food was boring, and eating "normally" was a lot more fun. Jane actually created her own boredom by the way in which she chose to think about her situation!

To avoid feeling bored and eventually backsliding again, Jane had to get control of her thinking and use positive self-talk in order to stay motivated about getting to goal weight. She also had to get herself interested in a project or activity separate from her weight control efforts, one that provided her with a sense of ongoing personal satisfaction.

Whenever possible, it is best to avoid a high risk situation altogether. Perhaps Mary Ann could have avoided the high risk situation of unexpectedly encountering tempting food if she had been more careful in cleaning out her pantry in the first place. But when it isn't possible to avoid a high risk situation, it is important to anticipate it, and to plan how to cope with it when it does occur.

Having a health problem interfere with being able to exercise is a common problem. If Susan had anticipated this possibility, and prepared herself in advance to cope with it, she might have returned to her exercise class once her cold was gone. She needed to have a plan ready for getting started again.

Sometimes, however, a high risk situation cannot be easily anticipated—but it is still possible to cope effectively. When Wilma's husband hurt his back, her obligations suddenly escalated, as did her stress level. Rather than taking on the additional burden herself, however, Wilma might have sought help from family or friends, perhaps getting a baby-sitter to allow her some personal time.

She actually needed her exercise more than ever, to keep her stress under control; and she could have used relaxation and deep breathing techniques as well. If she had understood how backsliding is triggered, and what she could do to cope more effectively with difficult situations, she would have been less likely to backslide.

Mary Ann could also have been prepared to cope. When she found the forgotten candy, she could have been ready and immediately tossed it in the garbage, reminding herself that she was doing so well managing her eating and that eating the candy wasn't worth the consequences. Had she done this, her self-confidence in her ability to take charge of her behavior would have increased, and the probability of backsliding would have decreased.

Instead, Mary Ann thought about how good the candy would taste, and rationalized that she would have "just one." But having eaten one piece and enjoyed it, she developed "tunnel vision." All she could see or think of was eating the rest of the candy, and any thoughts about managing her weight vanished.

After finishing the last bite and getting rid of the empty candy box so no one would know, Mary Ann started feeling guilty and angry with herself for blowing it. Filled with remorse, she decided there really wasn't any point in trying to control her eating because obviously she wasn't able to do so. This decision triggered another eating binge that lasted several days, together with more guilt and self-hate.

Having encountered a high risk situation and being unprepared to cope (or knowing what to do but not doing it), Mary Ann was unwittingly drawn into backsliding. In the process she experienced all of the hallmarks of the backsliding experience—encountering a high risk situation, not knowing what to do to cope (or knowing but not doing it), loss of self-confidence, tunnel vision, a first slip, guilt and self-blame, rationalizations and excuses, and finally collapse of all resolve and commitment.

Coping With High Risk Situations

To overcome backsliding that is triggered by a high risk situation, there are several things you should do:

1. *Learn to identify the high risk situations that may cause you difficulty.* Later in this chapter you will find a self-test, *What Makes You Backslide?* (page 227), which will help you identify your high risk situations. Take steps to avoid those that can be avoided. For those that cannot be avoided, try to anticipate possible problems and plan ahead how to cope more effectively— be prepared with some fall-back strategies.

2. *Be prepared with a coping response.* Know what to do. Mentally remind yourself of your commitment and why you made it. Tell yourself what to do to cope—then take positive action.

In Mary Ann's case, effective self-talk that would have helped her cope might have sounded like this: "Whoops! Where did this candy come from? Who knows, but I better get rid of it right now before I think any more about it. No, I won't have just one. That's a sure-fire way to risk backsliding. Quick. Grind up the candy in the disposal . . . Great, you did it. See. You can stay in control. You're on your way, girl. You can even handle booby traps like this!"

Such a coping response would have involved both thoughts and actions. If your thoughts start to slip into excuses and rationalizations, use thought stopping ("No, I won't let myself think that way"), and switch immediately to thoughts that help you cope ("How can I handle this effectively?"). Be willing to take drastic action if necessary—like tossing the candy in the disposal (instead of rationalizing that you'll save it for the kids).

3. *If you know you will have to deal with a high risk situation, use mental rehearsal to prepare for it.* Helen had learned that going out to lunch with a friend was a high risk situation for her. If the friend ordered a glass of wine or rich food, Helen would too. With mental rehearsal, she became better able to cope with the temptation.

Several times before meeting her friend for lunch, Helen would imagine the scene and see herself coping successfully. She would imagine her friend ordering a glass of wine and herself ordering a glass of mineral water. Then she would "see" her friend ordering something high in calories and herself ordering a good alternative. She even rehearsed how she would refuse if her friend urged her to order differently.

Most important of all, Helen would imagine feeling good about these decisions and having her confidence increase. Throughout the mental rehearsal and the actual event, she kept reminding herself that she was in control, and still enjoying herself.

Never let yourself encounter a high risk situation that you can anticipate without having mentally prepared for it. The best approach is to mentally imagine yourself handling the situation effectively and feeling good about it.

At the very least, decide in advance how you will cope. Plan ahead. Know in advance what you will order in a restaurant. Plan how to say "no" nicely but firmly. Decide what action you will take to avoid backsliding.

4. *When appropriate, bring to bear specific skills or techniques for coping.* When Wilma's husband hurt his back, his lack of mobility made him more cranky than usual. His irritation, together with the added burden of taking care of him, made Wilma's life, as well as her weight management efforts, more difficult.

To cope with his misdirected hostility, she needed better conflict management skills, and to remind herself not to take his irritation personally. To manage her own emotional upset, she should have made sure to exercise, and found time to do some meditation, even though she now had more obligations than before.

When she found that things were getting to her, she could have done some quick relaxation and deep breathing. It would have been helpful if she had spoken up for herself occasionally and asked her husband to be more understanding and sensitive, rather than suffering her own frustration in silence.

To avoid backsliding, be prepared to use positive self-talk, exercise, meditation, relaxation, assertive communication, and any other skills or techniques that will help you cope more effectively.

5.   *Avoid "tunnel vision."* When you have "tunnel vision," by definition your vision gets narrow, and you focus only on the temptation—eating, drinking, not exercising—to the exclusion of the other factors, such as your health, gaining weight, sticking to your commitment, and so forth. With tunnel vision often comes rationalizations about why you should give up your efforts.

One trick for avoiding tunnel vision is to keep handy your *Benefits and Costs Analysis* form from Chapter 2 and refer to it when a high risk situation is at hand. Be on guard with your self-talk; stop yourself from talking yourself into giving up, and think positive, motivating thoughts. You need to remind yourself of the reasons for making the commitment you made, and the hard work you have put in to achieve progress.

6.   *Learn to recover from a "first slip."* If at all possible, it is better to avoid a first slip. Most people do not stop at "just one," and the chances of recovering from a first slip are quite slim. Even if you do manage to handle "just one" the first time, you may become overconfident and think you can always handle "just one." But a succession of "just ones" can set the stage for eventual full-blown backsliding.

If you do succumb to a first slip, this does not have to signal full-blown backsliding. Instead of getting down on yourself, focus on what you can learn from the experience so that it is less likely to happen again.

Another helpful tool for preventing or recovering from a first slip is to carry with you a "reminder card." Like the seat pocket card the airlines use to tell you what to do in an emergency, a reminder card tells you what to do in case of a threatened or actual first slip.

Use an index card and write on it a brief reminder of why you made the commitment to change. Also note what actions you should take to either avoid a first slip or to recover from a first slip if it happens. It's a good idea to include the name and phone number of a friend you could call for support and advice. Carry the card with you, and if you ever need it, use it!

Overcoming Errors in Thinking

When Susan caught a cold and missed several of her exercise classes, she thought to herself, "I shouldn't exercise when I'm not feeling well, so I'll just lay off for a while." But not feeling up to par dragged on for several weeks, and by then Susan was enjoying not having to make the effort to exercise. When she thought about exercising, she focused on the difficulty of making time for exercise, and how nice it was to have time to do other things, and she rationalized that she was still sick and "you shouldn't exercise when you're sick." It was many months before Susan owned up to the fact that she was no longer sick but still not exercising.

While it is true that exercising when ill is inadvisable, Susan used this as an excuse to prolong not exercising. It is not necessary to feel 100% recovered before exercising again, and in fact, getting back to exercise quickly may speed recovery.

It is important to wait until the severe stage of an illness has passed. (When in doubt, get a doctor's advice.) But Susan overgeneralized. She used the excuse of having a simple cold to avoid exercising for many weeks. She filtered out information about the importance of exercise, and ignored thoughts that might argue for a return to exercising. She fell into several "thinking traps" that can lead to backsliding.

When Wilma's husband hurt his back, Wilma took on the burden of making him more comfortable, while still tending to her other obligations. Because of her sense of being responsible for everyone's happiness and well-being, she put others' needs before her own. This, together with rigid ideas about the way a good wife and mother should be, led her to give up her weight management program. She excused herself for quitting, saying that she just couldn't find time right now to worry about weight management.

Errors in thinking are almost always at the heart of backsliding, and they always accompany ineffective coping with a high risk situation. In Chapter 3, *Learning to "Think Smart"*, you learned about "thinking traps." These are ways in which you systematically distort the information of your senses. These distortions are not dissimilar to "bugs" in a computer program; they are glitches in the processing of information that foul up the output.

Everyone falls into thinking traps now and then, and doing so is not cause for self-condemnation. Rather, it is important to learn to recognize when you are caught in one, and to take the steps necessary to get out of it— challenge beliefs that no longer work, change negative attitudes, use supportive self-talk, and manage arousal effectively.

Setting Up Your Own Relapse

By allowing yourself to fall into thinking traps, and by making mini-decisions that seem of little importance at the time but which turn out to be quite important, you set up your own relapse. You can cause yourself to backslide just by the way you think.

Helen had finally gotten to goal weight after many months of diet and exercise. She was feeling good about herself and glad to be getting on about the business of her life without having to go to her weight management classes.

Little by little, however, she was letting her eating and exercise habits slip. Now and then she would rationalize, "I'll have just one." She told herself that one little piece of chocolate cake or an extra martini or two really wouldn't make that much difference, especially because she was exercising. But she was also missing more and more of her exercise sessions, excusing herself with "I'll get to it tomorrow."

She tried not to notice what was happening with her eating and exercise habits, and she stopped weighing herself regularly. The possibility of regaining weight was something she didn't want to think about. Instead she thought about how she deserved to eat without worrying, after all the effort she had made. Besides, with all the hassles she had to put up with in her job and with her family, she deserved to be nice to herself.

Mentally, Helen was priming herself to backslide. In her thoughts she was talking herself into making little decisions (making it okay to miss an exercise session), and into doing "unimportant" things (buying ice cream "for guests"), all of which were drawing her into backsliding.

She was becoming more and more aware that her clothes weren't fitting well, and she finally got on a scale to check it out. Sure enough, she had gained over ten pounds. She realized she was backsliding fast and well on her way to regaining all 40 pounds she had lost. She felt she had to do something immediately. In her panic, she looked for a quick solution and made an appointment with a local "shot" doctor.

Faulty Decision-Making

Part of the thinking process involves making decisions about what to do. Sometimes the quality of your decision-making is poor, and this further compounds a problem. For some time Helen had managed to ignore the continuing deterioration of her eating and exercise habits. She had found ways to rationalize why it was okay to eat inappropriately or not exercise, and she wouldn't let herself think about the consequences.

Helen had chosen a faulty decision-making strategy known as *defensive avoidance*. A person who is using defensive avoidance may try to ignore the fact that the problem exists. Or she may procrastinate and delay taking appropriate action. A defensive avoider tends to blame others for the problem, to construct wishful rationalizations that make it okay to choose a less objectionable alternative, and to minimize the probable consequences.

Defensive avoidance often allows the problem to get worse, until it can no longer be ignored, at which point panic may instigate yet another faulty decision-making strategy, *hypervigilance*—characterized by searching frantically for a way out of the dilemma and impulsively seizing whatever solution seems to promise immediate relief.

A better approach to making decisions is to be sure that you are in touch with what's really happening. Be on your guard against any tendency to deny or distort feedback information. Helen provided a good example. Early on she closed her eyes to the facts; she denied that her eating and exercise habits were slipping.

Armed with a realistic view of things, you can decide first if there is a problem, and then what to do about it. A *vigilant* decision-maker takes care to obtain relevant and accurate information needed to make the decision, is careful not to distort the facts, and considers various alternatives before making a choice.

Faulty decision-making can be either a contributor to or a consequence of backsliding. Helen started the process of backsliding by getting caught in thinking traps and using self-talk inappropriately. Along the way, she made some mini-decisions which contributed further to her backsliding.

For a time she defensively avoided acknowledging what was happening. Then once she did admit it, she panicked, and her ability to think clearly was further impaired. A host of thinking errors contributed to Helen's backsliding.

Coping With Errors in Thinking

Thinking guides behavior, and to overcome backsliding it is necessary to take charge of your thinking.

1. *Challenge and change irrational beliefs and ways of thinking.* Avoid being a perfectionist or falling into other thinking traps. Be sure the goals you have set for yourself are reasonable. If you find yourself taking something personally, try to mentally "rise above" the situation and not take it all so seriously.

Review Chapter 3, *Learning To "Think Smart"*, and learn to identify the beliefs and thinking traps that may be causing you trouble. These same ones are probably at the heart of your backsliding as well.

2. *Monitor and manage your self-talk.* Listen to what you are saying to yourself. If you are using excuses and rationalizations to allow yourself to eat inappropriately or to let your exercise slip, confront yourself. Use thought stopping to interrupt the excuses and rationalizations, and talk to yourself about your long-term goals and intentions.

Review your *Benefits and Costs Analysis* form from Chapter 2 to remind yourself of the long-term benefits of managing weight and the long-term costs of not doing so successfully. If you are using a "reminder card" (see the earlier section in this chapter on *Dealing With High Risk Situations*), be sure it contains some counter-arguments you can use to cope with your typical excuses and rationalizations.

3. *Become a better decision maker.* Avoid getting caught in defensive avoidance or hypervigilant decision-making strategies. Don't ignore a prob-

lem until it gets out of hand, and don't make important decisions when you are upset or panicked. Gently but regularly monitor your actions and be sure you are seeing the true picture. (You needn't be compulsive about this; just appropriately vigilant.) Be sure you have good information with which to make decisions and take action.

Changing an Unsupportive Context

A year beforehand, Gwenn had lost 60 pounds, but now she was having trouble maintaining. She and her husband had started a new business, and money was tight. He was often upset, and he took out his irritation on Gwenn, blaming her for a variety of problems and criticizing her excessively. And as if this weren't enough stress, Gwenn's teenage son was involved with drugs and having problems at school.

The constant stress of Gwenn's life was making it most difficult for her to maintain her new eating behaviors. She was keeping up her exercise, which gave her a good excuse to get away from the tension at home, but once home she would fall back into her old strategy for coping with stress—snacking.

The "context" of Gwenn's life was not supporting the maintenance of healthy eating habits and, indeed, was actively contributing to a return to old habits. An unsupportive context is a special kind of high risk situation, because it is ongoing.

A variety of things contribute to the context in which change and the maintenance of change takes place. Other people make up an important part of the context. The nature and quality of your interactions with them will influence your thinking, your emotions, and your behavior.

The economic situation is another part of the context which influences your ability to maintain change. The degree to which you must cope with personal or physical limitations, including addiction, biochemical dependence, genetics, physical handicaps or the necessity of taking certain medications, is also part of the context.

Finally, your ability to produce the results you want and to avoid results you don't want is integral to the context of your life. All of these factors (and others) are part of the fabric of life, and sometimes that fabric is not strong enough to support new behavior patterns.

The context can either contribute to backsliding, or it can help ensure success. When the people in your life are supportive, when your relationships are nurturing (or at least not destructive), when there is an adequate level of economic security, when you are not constrained by outside forces, and when you have abilities commensurate with your needs and goals, you are likely to have a context that works—a context that supports change and the maintenance of change. Conversely, when the context of your life is not helping to maintain your new behavior patterns, you need to take whatever steps you can to create a context that works to support and encourage the maintenance of change.

Creating a Context That Works

Influencing the context of your life and creating one that works may seem like a monumental task. Gwenn was barely holding herself and her family together in order to cope day to day. Yet even in this apparently dire situation, there were things she could have done that over time could have influenced and changed the context of her life.

1.   *Learn to be more interpersonally effective.* One important aspect of becoming more effective in interpersonal relationships is to learn how to communicate assertively. Another is to learn how not to take things personally, especially other people's barbs and nastiness. Gwenn needed to learn conflict management skills for distancing herself from her husband's criticism.

Be sure to review Chapter 6, *Improving Your Relationships,* for suggestions on how to create better relationships. It could also be helpful to enroll in programs specifically aimed at helping you become more assertive or better able to manage conflict.

2.   *Take action to change your environment.* One way to handle a difficult situation is to get out of it (as suggested in Chapter 7, *Managing Painful Emotions*). When this is not a realistic option, it is important to identify the resources available to make the situation less noxious.

Gwenn might have started by calling her local crisis center and asking for their suggestions. Your county mental health department and similar agencies may be able to help. Often churches can provide pastoral counseling that may be of assistance. Once you begin asking, you are likely to find sources of assistance you didn't know existed.

3.   *Don't automatically buy your limitations.* While it is important to take into account your actual limitations, it is also important not to sell yourself short. It is probably unrealistic to think you can make the Olympics if you are over 35 and severely overweight, but don't use being over 35 and severely overweight as an excuse for never being able to do something special, like run a marathon. Challenge your preconceived limitations. They may not be as limiting as you thought, or they may be completely imaginary.

Gwenn felt helpless to do anything about her situation. It seemed that nothing she did made any improvement, and she doubted her own competence, as well as her physical attractiveness. She was convinced that she wasn't very smart, and that everything was her fault.

Finally, however, with some assistance Gwenn was able to see that the constant criticism from her husband had led her to buy into limitations that simply had no basis. Prior to starting the new business with her husband, she had been a well thought of research scientist with a demonstrated ability to get results. She frequently received compliments from friends on her figure as well as her warm, friendly spirit. The problem lay not in her limitations, but in the stress and economic strain of undertaking a risky project with a partner who dealt with his stress by blaming others.

Real limitations are part of the context; the limitations in your head come from thinking errors. Richard Bach wrote in his book, *Illusions*, "Argue for your limitations, and sure enough they're yours." Take real limitations into account in your planning, but don't let them (or imagined limitations) keep you stuck in a problem.

4.   *Use a problem solving approach.* Sometimes you may make a valiant effort, and still not get the results you want. Perhaps you get no results at all, or you get results you hadn't expected. You might undertake a particular weight reduction method, following it as recommended, only to discover that you are not losing weight, or worse, you are gaining. When something like this happens, don't automatically blame yourself. It may be that the weight reduction method you have chosen is inadequate.

Instead of throwing up your hands and giving up all efforts to manage weight, take a problem solving approach. Ask yourself, "What is the real problem here? Is it a failure on my part, or a failure on the part of the method, or both?" Try to determine how your context may be working against you, instead of assuming the problem is entirely with you. If necessary, get professional advice. Use a vigilant decision-making strategy to decide what to do next.

Problem solving involves assuming that there is a problem and that there are a variety of solutions. You need only find the solution that is best for you. After gathering the facts, generate a number of possible solutions. Initially don't try to decide which is "best." After you have identified several possible solutions, choose one to try. Try it, and give it a chance to work. Then if necessary, try another one, and another one, until you get the results you desire, or until you must go back and reanalyze the problem, starting again from the beginning.

Developing Self-Management Skills

Many kinds of skills are needed to be successful in managing weight, as well as in living life effectively. Self-management skills involve learning how to identify and change your behavior patterns.

An important self-management tool is *self-monitoring*, which involves systematically gathering information on your perception of a particular problem, and tracking your progress in coping more effectively.

Self-management draws upon your skills in *problem solving*, because it requires being able to assess a problem, generate solution alternatives, establish a plan of action, and then try it out. Regularly assessing progress and revising strategy when necessary is an integral part of these skills. You need to be able to recover from a slip or temporary lapse, and renew your behavior change efforts.

Learning to *communicate effectively* is important in order to make relationships work. Skill in communicating assertively involves acknowledging and accepting your right to have your needs met, and your right to say "no" when someone else wants something from you. In the long run, relationships work better when you are willing to communicate openly, honestly, and without blaming. Effective listening is a complementary skill to communicating assertively.

Conflict is an inevitable part of interpersonal relationships, and the ability to *manage conflict* effectively when it does occur makes relationships healthier and more enjoyable. Often people who can't handle conflict retreat into themselves. They may have difficulty with intimacy, and may find it hard to make friends. Managing conflict and being able to create satisfying relationships are all vital skills for creating long-term success and happiness.

Another set of important skills involves *"thinking smart," coping with emotions,* and *managing stress effectively*. By learning to "think smart"— recognize and avoid thinking traps, challenge irrational beliefs, use your imagination effectively, and substitute encouraging self-talk for sabotaging self-talk—you are much more likely to avoid upsetting emotions.

But sometimes feeling bad is unavoidable. It may be an understandable reaction to difficult circumstances or life problems. You need to be able to recognize the difference between healthy and unhealthy emotions. When painful emotions do occur, you need to know how to use stress management techniques and other techniques—such as meditation, deep breathing, thought stopping, exercise, and so forth—for coping more effectively.

A related skill that helps minimize stress is *time management*—knowing how to identify the tasks that need to be done, by creating a "to do" list, setting priorities, deciding which tasks need the most attention, and then structuring your day so that the important tasks are handled first. This involves creating and following a plan of action. An important part of avoiding stress from time pressures is to notice and acknowledge your accomplishments at the end of the day, and to avoid undertaking more obligations than you can reasonably handle.

Rate your level of skills in each of these areas according to whether you need to acquire certain skills, whether you need more practice in doing what you already know how to do, or whether you already have good skills.

Self-Test 10.1

Skills Assessment

	Need to acquire	Need more practice	Good Skills
1. *Self-Management Skills*—The ability to gather information to help you understand your behavior and manage environmental influences to gain greater control over behavior.	____	____	____
2. *Problem Solving Skills*—The ability to assess the problem inherent in a difficult situation, generate solution alternatives, and try out various alternatives until a satisfactory solution is found.	____	____	____
3. *Skill in Getting Remotivated*—The ability to recover from a first slip or from an interruption of effort and to get started again.	____	____	____
4. *Skill in Communicating Assertively*—The ability to communicate in such a way that you get your needs met while respecting the rights of others, including the ability to say "no" when appropriate.	____	____	____
5. *Conflict Management Skills*—The ability to minimize and when necessary cope with interpersonal anger and disagreement.	____	____	____
6. *Skill in Initiating or Maintaining Social Relationships*—The ability to make and keep friends.	____	____	____
7. *Thinking Skills*—The ability to minimize errors in thinking, challenge irrational beliefs, use imagery, and substitute encouraging self-talk for self-defeating thoughts.	____	____	____
8. *Skill in Coping with Emotions*—The ability to distinguish between healthy and unhealthy emotional reactions to difficult situations or life problems and take appropriate steps to cope.	____	____	____
9. *Stress Management Skills*—The ability to elicit the relaxation response to cope with physical arousal.	____	____	____
10. *Time Management Skills*—The ability to identify tasks, set priorities, structure your day, and stay focused on your plan of action.	____	____	____

Acquiring Better Skills

Self-management and problem solving skills, as well as skills in thinking and coping with emotions, are necessary for long-term weight management success. You may feel the need for more in-depth work in some skill areas, such as communicating assertively, managing conflict, relating better to others, managing time, and using meditation or other stress management techniques.

Where you feel the need for more in-depth work, investigate the availability of classes or programs in your area, or obtain self-help books or other materials that might assist you.

For those skill areas you checked as "need to acquire" in the *Skills Assessment* self-test, go back and review the appropriate chapters in this book. For those skill areas you rated "need more practice," set some performance goals (number of times per day or week that you will do something), and then keep track of your progress.

Getting Your Lifestyle in Balance

Lifestyle can be yet another major cause of backsliding. Maggie joined a weight control program when she found herself increasingly upset over her slow, steady weight gain. She was sure that her weight was keeping her from finding a satisfactory, romantic relationship, and she said that life as a single person just wasn't much fun any more.

Upon joining the weight control program, Maggie indicated to the facilitator that she would have to miss several meetings because she traveled extensively in her work, but she was adamant about her commitment to complete the program and lose weight.

However, when she returned to class the second session, Maggie reported she had misplaced the previous week's handouts, and as a result had not read the material for the present session or started the self-monitoring of her eating habits. The following week she complained that keeping records was too much of a hassle, especially since she had to do that all day long in her job.

Furthermore, she couldn't see how she could start an exercise program because she rose for work at 6:00 a.m., used lunch time for business, and stayed late at work. She didn't have time to eat breakfast and get to work on time, so she just gulped a cup of coffee and smoked a cigarette in the car. Coffee and cigarettes were her main sustenance during the day, except for a big "business" lunch, with a glass of wine or two. By the time she got home in the evening, she was too exhausted to do anything more than pour herself a drink and grab something quick to eat from the freezer.

Maggie missed the fourth meeting of her program because she had to go out of town on business. When she returned for the fifth meeting, she was discouraged because she showed a gain of two pounds. She never returned to another meeting. An unbalanced lifestyle had caused Maggie to backslide by dropping out and relinquishing her commitment.

A balanced lifestyle is one that has a relative degree of balance between those things you must do (and that are potential sources of stress), and the things you want to do (and that make life pleasant). An unbalanced lifestyle is one characterized by too many "shoulds" and not enough "wants." There is more work than play, more obligations than rewards. Energy is directed outward, with little time or energy left for activities that give personal pleasure, satisfaction, or self-fulfillment.

When your lifestyle is unbalanced, you are likely to feel deprived, with a periodic need for self-indulgence. The probability of backsliding is very high, unless something is done to bring more balance into the lifestyle by reducing obligations and/or increasing the opportunities for reward and nurturing.

Stress in life can come from major life events, such as divorce, illness, loss of employment, or the death of a loved one, or it can come from ongoing daily hassles. Although traumatic life events can be the source of considerable stress, in terms of health, and for long-term success in weight management, the ability to handle day-to-day stress is more important.

If you have an unbalanced lifestyle, you may be attempting to cope with the attendant stress by engaging in one or more "negative" addictions—abuse of alcohol, smoking cigarettes, drinking excessive amounts of caffeine, or inappropriate eating. Engaging in such behaviors is an attempt to restore some balance and to nurture yourself as well as to reduce the physical overstimulation that comes with stress.

Assessing Your Lifestyle

Perhaps you are already aware that yours is an unbalanced lifestyle. Or perhaps, like Maggie, you are so caught up in it that you don't recognize how the way you have your life setup is the underlying cause of more problems than just your weight. If you are not sure about the balance between "shoulds" and "wants" in your life, you need to find out if there is a problem. The following self-monitoring exercise will help you do this.

Self-Monitoring Your Daily Activities

For several days or a week, record your daily activities using the *Want To/Have To Inventory* form given on page 220. Indicate those that are obligations and those that you choose to do for yourself, by rating each activity as a "want to"

Want To/Have To Inventory

Activity	Want To	Mixture	Have To	Satisfaction		
				High	Med	Low

Want To/Have To Assessment

Number of "Want To"
Activities that are: _____ High in satisfaction

_____ Medium in satisfaction

_____ Low in satisfaction

_____ **Total "Want To" Activities**

Number of "Mixture"
Activities that are: _____ High in satisfaction

_____ Medium in satisfaction

_____ Low in satisfaction

_____ **Total "Mixture" Activities**

Number of "Have To"
Activities that are: _____ High in satisfaction

_____ Medium in satisfaction

_____ Low in satisfaction

_____ **Total "Have To" Activities**

(an activity you aren't obligated to do but which you choose to do), a "mixture" (of want to and have to), or a "have to" (an activity that is an obligation, whether or not you like doing it).

Then rate the degree of pleasure, satisfaction, or self-fulfillment you get from each—high, medium, or low. At the end of each day, total the number of "want to" activities according to the degree of satisfaction they yield, the number of "mixture" activities according to the degree of satisfaction they yield, and the number of "have to" activities and the degree of satisfaction they yield.

If you have more "have to" than "want to" activities, you may have a lifestyle that is unbalanced. Look at the totals, together with your satisfaction ratings. What degree of satisfaction are the activities yielding? If you have given high satisfaction ratings to the "have to" activities, and few to the "want to" activities, or if almost all of your activities are a "mixture," you may still have an unbalanced lifestyle.

People who are hard-driving and achievement-oriented often get more satisfaction from their jobs than from their personal lives. They become workaholics, and often suffer high degrees of stress, because they fill their lives with "have to's" and find it difficult to make time for "want to's" (which they often regard as frivolous and unproductive). Even when engaging in "want to" activities, their minds may be on "have to" activities. Their unbalanced lifestyle leaves little time for real relaxation and self-nurturing.

If you have a high number of "have to" or "mixture" activities relative to "want to" activities, and your satisfaction ratings are predominantly "medium" or "low," you are probably quite aware that you are leading an unbalanced lifestyle. Another indicator that your lifestyle is unbalanced is the presence of negative addictions—drinking, smoking, overeating, gambling, excessive spending.

By definition, an unbalanced lifestyle is one that is unsatisfactory in some or all aspects. Maggie knew that there was a problem somewhere because her experience of life was not complete. She decided that losing weight was the answer. In fact, weight was not the main problem but the result of the main problem. Maggie had taken on so many obligations at work that she had little or no time to nurture herself.

While Maggie's job gave her prestige and a high salary, it also cost her dearly. The rewards of the job kept her handcuffed to undertaking excessive obligations. Until she is ready to reassess her priorities in life, and make some changes in her present level of obligations, successful weight management will be illusive.

Situations such as Maggie's prompt many people to seek the quick fix, the easy answer, the latest diet or miracle cure for weight, rather than to undertake the steps that will ensure lifelong success in managing weight— and that often includes creating a more balanced lifestyle.

Restoring Balance to Your Lifestyle

Restoring balance to an unbalanced lifestyle begins with an assessment of current ways of coping. What are the strategies you use now to cope with the hassles of daily life? Place a check mark by all of the following "negative" addictions or inappropriate ways of coping with stress that apply to you:

Negative Addictions

____ eating inappropriately, including snacking, skipping meals, eating the wrong foods, overeating

____ smoking, including using marijuana, to relieve stress or obtain pleasure

____ using alcohol to excess or to cope with stress, tension, or unpleasant emotions

____ using unprescribed drugs or abusing prescribed drugs to deal with stress

____ sleeping too much, including napping or dozing without cause

____ overcharging with credit cards or spending beyond your means

____ gambling, betting, playing cards or bingo to excess

____ watching TV to excess

Having identified your negative coping styles, decide how you will tackle and change them. Where shall you begin? What kind of assistance will you need? What positive coping styles do you need to integrate into your life?

A balanced lifestyle is characterized by certain "positive" addictions and appropriate coping strategies:

Positive Addictions

1. Eating a healthy, low-fat, high-complex-carbohydrate diet.

2. Regularly engaging in a well-rounded program of exercise.

3. Getting adequate relaxation and personal satisfaction by engaging in sufficient "want to" activities.

4. Having satisfying social contacts and engaging in interpersonal activities that provide a sense of acceptance and connectedness.

5. Having a life philosophy or spiritual grounding that provides guidance for life decisions.

Assessing Your "Want To" Activities

To restore balance to your lifestyle, you also need to identify "want to" activities, and plan to include more of them in your life. It's not healthy spending most of your time doing what you don't really like to do, or only what you must do. It is important to do things that nurture or "give back" energy to you. By completing the *20 Things I Love To Do* worksheet located on page 225 (sample on page 224), you can explore what activities do this for you, and perhaps begin to discover what it is you really want out of life.

First, list 20 things you love to do. They can be big or little things in your life; things appealing to the senses, or more abstract pleasures; things you've always enjoyed, or relatively new experiences; things that you do, or that others do for you; things done indoors or outdoors, at night or during the day, or in different seasons of the year.

Be as specific as possible. Instead of just listing "sports," write "watching Monday night football on TV," or "playing tennis with my partner." Put

Self-Test 10.2

Sample   *20 Things I Love to Do*

Activity:	$	A–P	PL	N5	1–5	Days
1. sketching		A	PL			
2. walking through buildings and looking at architecture		A	PL			
3. hiking		A/P	PL			
4. going to the movies	$	A/P	PL		3.	2
5. playing with my dog		A			1.	0
6. going to the beach		P	PL			
7. reading fun stuff		A			2.	1
8. watching TV news		A			4.	3
9. having friends over		P	PL		5.	1 mo.
10. sitting in a hot tub		P	PL			
11. getting a massage		P	PL	N5		
12. giving a massage		P	PL	N5		
13. talking to Claudia on the phone		P				
14. trying out new recipes	$	A	PL			
15.						
16.						
17.						
18.						
19.						
20.						

Source: M. McKay, M. Davis, and P. Fanning, *Thoughts and Feelings: The Art of Cognitive Stress Intervention,* New Harbinger Publications, Oakland, CA, 1981. Used with permission.

Self-Test 10.2

20 Things I Love to Do

Activity:	$	A–P	PL	N5	1–5	Days
1. _____						
2. _____						
3. _____						
4. _____						
5. _____						
6. _____						
7. _____						
8. _____						
9. _____						
10. _____						
11. _____						
12. _____						
13. _____						
14. _____						
15. _____						
16. _____						
17. _____						
18. _____						
19. _____						
20. _____						

Source: M. McKay, M. Davis, and P. Fanning, *Thoughts and Feelings: The Art of Cognitive Stress Intervention,* New Harbinger Publications, Oakland, CA, 1981. Used with permission.

down on the list whatever comes to your mind, without judging it or wondering what others might think. You may have a few more or a few less than 20 items. Then, after getting all your items down on the list, use the adjacent rating grid to indicate certain characteristics of each activity you love to do.

If it costs over $5 each time you do it, put a "$" in the first column. If you like to do it alone, write an "A" in the next column, or if you do it with others, write a "P." If you like to do it alone or with others, write "A/P." If the activity requires planning, write "PL" in the third column. If you would not have listed this five years ago, write "N5" in the fourth column. In the fifth column, choose the five activities you love most, and rank them from 1 to 5 in order of preference. Finally, write approximately how many days it has been since you last engaged in each activity.

When you have finished, review this analysis of your "want to" activities. What does it suggest about why you experience the level of satisfaction in life that you do? How might your level of "want to" activities be related to your weight management efforts?

Perhaps you had difficulty thinking of many items to put on this list. Is this because you have forgotten what it is you like to do, or perhaps because you have never taken that much time for yourself?

Some people find this exercise very upsetting, because they realize how little they actually do for themselves. The purpose of the exercise is to bring you face to face with this possibility, so that if you have not been nurturing yourself sufficiently, you can create and integrate more "want to" activities into your lifestyle.

What Makes You Backslide?

Many things can contribute to backsliding. Encountering a "high risk" situation and not having a coping response ready is one. The probability is further increased when there are errors in thinking. Not knowing how to recover from a slip also increases the chances of full-scale backsliding.

Sometimes, however, backsliding happens because the circumstances simply mediate against the maintenance of new behavior patterns. A variety of skills help ensure maintenance, including skills in communicating effectively, self-management skills, stress management skills, and interpersonal skills. However, when your lifestyle is characterized by too many obligations and not enough personal rewards, you will need to make some basic changes in your lifestyle, perhaps reordering priorities and taking care to nurture yourself adequately.

To overcome backsliding you need to determine what makes you backslide. Complete the *What Makes You Backslide?* self-test to help you do this. Armed with this information, you can adopt an effective plan of action.

(text continues on page 230)

Self-Test 10.3

What Makes You Backslide?

Indicate the extent to which each of the following situations is likely to cause you to backslide—to relinquish your commitment to change your eating or exercise behavior and return to bad habits. Circle "0" if the situation is "not applicable"; that is, it doesn't happen to you. For situations that do happen to you, use the rating scale and give a low rating ("1" or "2") if the situation is less likely to cause you to backslide. Give a higher rating ("4" or "5") if a situation is more likely to cause you to backslide. (Hint: To help you in rating each situation, recall previous times when you have made a similar commitment to change and then backslid. Circle *one number only* for each situation.)

Rating   1—Not likely to cause me to backslide.
2—Somewhat likely to cause me to backslide.
3—Could go either way.
4—Somewhat likely to cause me to backslide.
5—Highly likely to cause me to backslide.

	N/A	Least Likely			Most Likely	
1. You feel frustrated, annoyed, or angry.	0	1	2	3	4	5
2. You feel worried, apprehensive, anxious, or afraid.	0	1	2	3	4	5
3. You feel sad or depressed.	0	1	2	3	4	5
4. You feel alone, empty, or lonely.	0	1	2	3	4	5
5. You feel tense or under stress.	0	1	2	3	4	5
6. You get bored or restless.	0	1	2	3	4	5
7. You feel shy or intimidated.	0	1	2	3	4	5
8. You are suffering from pain, illness, or injury.	0	1	2	3	4	5
9. You feel tired, fatigued, or exhausted.	0	1	2	3	4	5
10. You experience negative effects from medications you are taking.	0	1	2	3	4	5
11. You feel shaky, lightheaded, or nauseous.	0	1	2	3	4	5
12. You feel jumpy, nervous, or irritable.	0	1	2	3	4	5
13. You are having fun or feeling "high."	0	1	2	3	4	5
14. You are relaxing.	0	1	2	3	4	5
15. You are feeling secure, accepted, or loved.	0	1	2	3	4	5
16. You are enjoying yourself.	0	1	2	3	4	5
17. You think you can handle "just one."	0	1	2	3	4	5
18. You want to test your willpower or ability to cope with temptation.	0	1	2	3	4	5
19. You decide you've "got it knocked" and let down a little bit.	0	1	2	3	4	5

(continued)

Self-Test 10.3

What Makes You Backslide? (continued)

	N/A	*Least Likely*			*Most Likely*	
20. You feel you can handle things without any more help.	0	1	2	3	4	5
21. You have a sudden inclination to give in to a temptation.	0	1	2	3	4	5
22. You experience an enduring or recurring desire for something that was part of the old behavior pattern.	0	1	2	3	4	5
23. You feel a compulsion for something that you now regard as "off limits."	0	1	2	3	4	5
24. You have a craving for something.	0	1	2	3	4	5
25. You get into an argument or disagreement with someone.	0	1	2	3	4	5
26. Someone takes advantage of you or hurts your feelings.	0	1	2	3	4	5
27. You feel hassled or "put upon" by someone.	0	1	2	3	4	5
28. Someone exhibits jealousy towards you.	0	1	2	3	4	5
29. Someone puts you down or is highly critical of you.	0	1	2	3	4	5
30. You feel "closed out" by someone.	0	1	2	3	4	5
31. Someone wants you to give up your commitment to lose weight or get fit.	0	1	2	3	4	5
32. You see others eating.	0	1	2	3	4	5
33. Someone gives you a gift of food or brings something to eat especially for you.	0	1	2	3	4	5
34. Others do things that undermine your efforts to lose weight or exercise.	0	1	2	3	4	5
35. You are celebrating or having a good time with others.	0	1	2	3	4	5
36. You are enjoying togetherness or comradeship.	0	1	2	3	4	5
37. You are experiencing good feelings with someone.	0	1	2	3	4	5
38. You are feeling good in a social situation.	0	1	2	3	4	5
39. You aren't getting the results you want.	0	1	2	3	4	5

Scoring

The situations you rated either a "4" or "5" are those most likely to cause you to backslide. These situations are grouped by type of cause under the heading *Causes of Backsliding* listed in the box on page 230.

To determine where you need to focus your efforts, tally the number of situations in each group of *Situations* that you rated a "4" or "5" and put this number in the column, *No. of Situations Rated "4" or "5."* Then multiply that

Self-Test 10.3

What Makes You Backslide? (continued)

	N/A	Least Likely			Most Likely	
40. You question how important losing weight or getting fit really is to you.	0	1	2	3	4	5
41. You keep remembering how you've tried before and didn't succeed.	0	1	2	3	4	5
42. You keep thinking you "can't" or that it's "too hard."	0	1	2	3	4	5
43. You won't let yourself think about your increasing number of eating indiscretions, or how long it's been since you've exercised.	0	1	2	3	4	5
44. You are experiencing concerns about money.	0	1	2	3	4	5
45. You are having marital problems.	0	1	2	3	4	5
46. Your family or cultural group has different ideas about what's good for you.	0	1	2	3	4	5
47. You have physical limitations.	0	1	2	3	4	5
48. You are feeling overwhelmed.	0	1	2	3	4	5
49. When confronted with temptation, you don't know how to cope.	0	1	2	3	4	5
50. You have time pressures or deadlines to meet.	0	1	2	3	4	5
51. You get through a crisis okay until afterwards.	0	1	2	3	4	5
52. An unexpected crisis occurs.	0	1	2	3	4	5
53. You do everything you are supposed to do but it isn't working, so you give up.	0	1	2	3	4	5
54. The stress in your life gets out of hand.	0	1	2	3	4	5
55. You feel the need to nurture yourself.	0	1	2	3	4	5
56. You want to make yourself feel good.	0	1	2	3	4	5
57. You want relief from the press of your obligations.	0	1	2	3	4	5
58. You don't have time for yourself.	0	1	2	3	4	5
59. You don't have enough time for family or social activities.	0	1	2	3	4	5

number by the adjacent correction factor, rounding off to the nearest whole number. Put this corrected score in the *Score* column.

Then look at the *Score* column. The highest possible score for any one *Cause of Backsliding* is "4." The groupings that you have the highest scores in are the ones that you need to focus on. After determining which *Causes of Backsliding* present a problem for you, review the material in this chapter for specific suggestions on dealing with that type of cause.

Causes of Backsliding	Situations:	No. of Situations Rated "4" or "5":	Correction Factor:	Score
Negative Emotions and Moods	1–7	_____	x .6	_____
Negative Physical States	8–13	_____	x .7	_____
Private Positive Emotions	14–17	_____	x 1.0	_____
Test of Personal Control	18–21	_____	x 1.0	_____
Urges or Temptations	22–25	_____	x 1.0	_____
Interpersonal Conflict	26–31	_____	x .7	_____
Social Influences	32–35	_____	x 1.0	_____
Interpersonal Positive Emotions	36–39	_____	x 1.0	_____
Errors in Thinking	40–44	_____	x .8	_____
Unsupportive Context	45–48	_____	x 1.0	_____
Lack of Skills	49–55	_____	x .6	_____
Unbalanced Lifestyle	56–59	_____	x .8	_____

This may involve learning how to anticipate and cope with high risk situations, changing your way of thinking, attempting to create a more supportive context for the maintenance of change, acquiring and using new skills, and bringing more balance into your lifestyle.

Summary

Many things can trigger backsliding—including high risk and crisis situations, errors in thinking, unsupportive context, skills deficits, and an unbalanced lifestyle.

To overcome backsliding, it is necessary to develop skills for coping with these factors. An important place to begin is to discover what particular factors cause you to backslide. When you have identified these, you can choose the best solution to avoid, change, or cope better with problematic situations.

References

1. Marlatt, G.A., & Gordon, J.R. (1985). *Relapse Prevention*. New York: Guilford.

2. Grilo, C.M., Shiffman, S., & Wing, R.R. (1989). Relapse crises and coping among dieters. *Journal of Consulting and Clinical Psychology, 57,* 488–495.

Chapter 11

Reaching Out
For Help

ONE OF THE EXPLANATIONS Oprah gave for regaining weight was that she didn't feel comfortable talking in group therapy about her childhood sexual abuse, so she dropped out. She has recently declared her intention to speak out against such abuse, perhaps as a means of healing her own childhood trauma. For many others who have been the victims of abuse, therapy has been the avenue for coming to terms with the experience.

More and more women are coming forward, both in therapy and in the media, to talk about childhood experiences that have severely limited their ability to experience adult life in a satisfactory manner. Roseanne Barr Arnold has made appearances before live audiences, as well as on television talk shows, to make public her incest experience, which she has also dealt with in individual therapy.

Clinicians who work with women who are seriously overweight, as Oprah and Roseanne both are, are familiar with how frequently sexual, physical, and emotional abuse are in the backgrounds of these women. Often, women with serious weight problems suffer from depression, anxiety, and a variety of other psychological afflictions. When these problems are significant, as they are with such abuse, or when the normal course of time does not heal the sufferer, it is time to seek professional help.

As strange as it may seem, there are still some people who don't seek therapy because they are too embarrassed or ashamed. They think that a person who wants therapy must be "crazy" or "sick." It is often hard for such a person to reach out for help, because she is so invested in being seen by others, as well as by herself, as being in control and "having it together."

Still other people resent having to pay someone to "just sit there and listen." Why not talk to a friend? Or they believe you should just forget what troubles you and get on with life.

As Robert Langs, M.D., states in his book, *Rating Your Psychotherapist*, psychotherapy is a peculiarly intimate personal experience.[1] The patient entrusts his or her most deeply felt secrets to a stranger, who in turn commits his or her own interest and concern—and expertise—to another's experience of pain and confusion. Together they work toward the patient's greater self-awareness, maturity, and healing.

Dr. Jerome D. Frank of Johns Hopkins University Medical School notes that psychotherapy "is a planned, emotionally charged, confiding interaction between a trained, socially-sanctioned healer and a sufferer."[2] The primary vehicle for healing is words, though sometimes bodily activities are involved. In some cases, the patient's relatives and others may be included in the process. Dr. Frank asserts that the aim of all psychotherapy is to help the person accept and endure suffering as an inevitable aspect of life, and to use it as an opportunity for personal growth.

The most valuable thing the therapist brings to therapy, in addition to extensive training and practice, is that he or she is an *objective third party*. As such, the therapist can listen with a dispassionate ear and provide a relatively unbiased perspective that a friend or untrained person could not. In addition, the therapist's suggestions and insights come from informed study of the field of human behavior.

The fact that psychotherapy is a service for which a fee is charged ensures that a time and a place are bracketed off for this activity. This in part is what establishes the therapeutic relationship as different from a friendship or from the sharing of problems with a neighbor. In addition, unlike talking to friends or family, the therapeutic relationship is more likely to be a safe place to talk confidentially about disturbing issues without being judged or made to feel wrong.

Finding a Therapist

Even though a person may come to realize that she could benefit from therapy, she may not know how to go about finding a psychotherapist, or what to expect once she has found one.

There are many ways to find a therapist. Probably the best way is to ask someone you trust, preferably a professional, to give you several names of therapists you might consider. It is preferable to get two or three names from the same person and ask that referral source to indicate how the therapists who are being recommended differ from each other.

Physicians, other therapists, mental health practitioners, nurses, religious leaders, school or job counselors, are all good sources for getting names of potential therapists. It could also be helpful to ask for a referral from a friend or a relative whose contact with a therapist is professional and non-personal—that is, that person does not have a present therapeutic relationship with the therapist.

It is better not to get a referral from someone who is presently a patient of the therapist, because this relationship might unconsciously impair your trust of the therapist. Although this kind of source might seem to offer the advantage of first-hand experience with the therapist's approach, there are other, less risky ways to assess the suitability of a therapist. Rather than just going to a friend's therapist, take the time and make the effort to find your own.

It is decidedly not a good idea to get a referral from a public source, such as a book written by the therapist, a news article, or an appearance on radio or television. While in principle such professionals should be okay, assuming they are licensed, the "public figure" therapist may be more interested in fame and fortune than in your problems. In addition, you may bring expectations of his or her expertise to the therapy, as a result of the therapist's celebrity status, which could ultimately be counterproductive for your work together.

Likewise, getting a name from the telephone book, from an advertisement, or from seeing a shingle hung outside an office results in a potluck choice that may or may not meet your needs.

Definitely do not go to a therapist whom you know socially or whose personal life you know about. For example, this would include a therapist whose children are in the same class at school as your children, or who is your minister, or who is the wife or husband of a friend. Your having extensive knowledge of a therapist's personal life can get in the way of your therapy. (If you live in a small town, it may be more difficult to meet this condition. In such a case, you should at least discuss this concern with the prospective therapist.)

Differences Between Therapists

Understanding the differences in the therapeutic orientations of therapists and how a particular therapeutic orientation can be expected to affect your experience in therapy is useful in selecting a therapist. Most therapists are trained in or favor a certain school of thought, and this will affect the way in which he or she interacts with you. Different techniques, such as dream analysis, role playing, or homework may be used, depending on the therapist's orientation.

Be aware that anyone may call themself a "psychotherapist." This label gives no guarantee of any formal training or professional recognition. Even though most states have laws that make it illegal to represent oneself as a licensed "psychologist" or to practice psychology without a license, there are no laws against using the label "psychotherapist." This is a general term that does not imply a specific background or any credentials recognized by other mental health professionals. Similarly, such labels as hypnotherapist or massage therapist indicate no guarantee that the person using them has any formal training in psychology, psychiatry, or mental health.

In the past, most therapists were trained in one particular school of thought that made certain assumptions about the human behavior and the process of change. Each school believed its approach to be the best or "right" one, and rejected rival claims to efficacy.

More recently, observers of the field of psychotherapy are beginning to detect increasing signs that representatives of different schools are willing to acknowledge the potential value of a range of techniques and to show increasing flexibility in applying them. Proponents of different schools of thought have begun to explore their commonalities, as well as what they might profitably learn from one another.

As a result, many therapists are more willing to present themselves as "eclectic"—that is, although trained in one particular approach to psychotherapy, they are willing and able to adopt a different strategy, depending on the patient or the presenting problem.

Despite this move toward a more pragmatic psychotherapeutic strategy, the primary training and theoretical orientation of the therapist is likely to exert a significant influence. There are several main schools of thought that dictate the particular approach to psychotherapy a therapist may use: psychodynamic psychotherapy (of which, psychoanalysis is a subset), behavior therapy, cognitive therapy, cognitive-behavior therapy, humanistic and existential psychotherapy, and family systems approaches.

Psychodynamic Psychotherapy

Psychodynamic psychotherapy has become an umbrella term that includes a variety of schools of thought or theoretical orientations that have their origins in traditional *psychoanalytic theory*.

Psychoanalysis, which is the "grandfather" of all psychodynamic psychotherapy, is a system of psychology derived from the work of Sigmund Freud. The underlying premise of psychoanalysis is that the mind is the expression of conflicting forces, some of which are unconscious. The patient's early experiences and how she resolved certain major issues is thought to be critical.

In therapy attention is given to examining those early years, as well as to the analysis of defense mechanisms and resistance. Another subject for interpretation in psychoanalysis is the way in which the patient relates to the therapist, which is also seen as a reflection of earlier relationships.

The therapist tends to assume a neutral stance intended to help the patient gain insight into his relationships in the present and to work though conflicts. The therapist does not offer advice and avoids being directive. In traditional psychoanalysis, the patient comes to therapy more than once a week, and is expected to talk about whatever comes to mind. The analysis of this "free association," as well as of dreams, is the primary activity in this type of therapy. Therapy may last from 2 to 10 years or more.

Instead of assuming that conflict underlies functioning, newer psychodynamic schools of thought assume that a deficit, usually originating in childhood, affects current experience.

One of the more prominent, psychodynamic approaches that presumes a developmental deficit is based on *object relations theory*. Therapy from an object relations perspective takes as its focus problems people have in developing or sustaining gratifying relationships with others. Symptoms such as anxiety or depression are assumed to be the result of problems with interpersonal relationships that are threatening the patient's sense of self.

Difficulties the patient experiences in the world are expected to be repeated in the therapist-patient relationship. Thus, the therapist-patient relationship *itself* becomes a focus for change. In contrast to the psychoanalytic psychotherapist, the object relations therapist is more interactive and forthcoming. In object relations therapy, the therapist is more likely to comment on current interactions, including those with the therapist, than to focus on analyzing the past. The patient is more likely to experience the therapist as caring, committed, and involved.

Yet a different theoretical orientation that falls under the rubric of psychodynamic psychotherapy is that of Carl Jung's *analytical psychotherapy*. In Jungian therapy, the focus is on the meaning of symbols and the relationship between the conscious and the unconscious. Dreamwork is the core of this approach to therapy, and the therapist assists the patient to come to greater self-knowledge through the analysis of dreams and symbols as they present themselves in the patient's life.

In most psychodynamic psychotherapy, patients usually participate in therapy once a week in the therapist's office or clinic setting. Like psychoanalysis, psychodynamic psychotherapy is expected to be long-term, often lasting years.

Behavior Therapy

In contrast to psychodynamic approaches to therapy, the behavior therapist is not particularly interested in early experience and does not offer interpretations of past experiences for the sake of insight. Behaviorists pay little heed to the notion of unconscious forces or unobservable behaviors such as thoughts. The focus of behavior therapy is on learned behavior patterns, and the environmental factors that elicit or reinforce their occurrence in the here-and-now.

The behavior therapist focuses on defining the problem in terms of the specific environmental events that elicit the problematic behavior and the factors that sustain the behavior. Once the pattern is understood, specific techniques are chosen for intervening to change the pattern. The therapist is active and directive, designing interventions and making suggestions. Depending on the presenting problem, the therapy may take place outside the therapist's office. For example, the therapist may go on an airplane trip with a client who is afraid of flying.

The client (behaviorists do not use the term "patient") is usually given specific tasks to complete between sessions, and is expected to participate actively in carrying out the change techniques. The client may be taught to use such techniques as self-monitoring (i.e., counting instances of a specific behavior), relaxation, and behavior rehearsal.

The hallmark of behavior therapy is its reliance on techniques and interventions that have been shown by research to work. The types of problems that behavioral approaches tend to address include lack of assertiveness, anxiety and phobias, habit and lifestyle problems such as smoking and overeating.

Behavioral therapy takes no longer than the time necessary to relieve the symptoms. This may take as little as one session. More often it lasts from 10 to 20 sessions.

Cognitive Therapy

The basic premise of cognitive therapy is that how one thinks largely determines how one feels and behaves. The therapy is a collaborative process between therapist and client, and focuses primarily on correcting faulty information processing through identifying and changing distortions in thinking, irrational beliefs, and self-talk. Interventions include keeping a record of thoughts, developing counterarguments for negative thoughts and beliefs, and learning to use self-instructional thoughts to cope with stressful situations.

Cognitive therapy has been shown to be particularly helpful for depression, especially if the depressive symptoms are generated by negative thinking. Clients are expected to do homework between sessions that might include self-monitoring of thoughts and taking specific steps to change thinking. Symptoms are often relieved in 10 to 20 sessions.

Cognitive-Behavior Therapy

Cognitive-behavior therapy is a blend of behavior therapy and cognitive therapy. Both the behavioral and the cognitive or thinking components that contribute to a problem are identified, and these become the focus for intervention. In addition, skills training is an important aspect of dealing with the overall problem. A number of problems, including obesity, smoking, stress management, and pain management, have been found to be successfully treated with cognitive-behavior interventions.

Like behavior therapy and cognitive therapy, the duration of therapy usually depends on symptom relief. However, there is a recent move toward providing longer-term therapy for more chronic problems such as obesity and personality problems.

Humanistic/Existential Approaches

Although less popular today than previously, therapy based on humanistic and/or existential assumptions is still utilized by many therapists.

Carl Roger's person-centered therapy is the prototypic example of the humanistic approach in individual therapy. The basis of this approach is to promote trust so that the client will become self-actualized—that is, become "fully human" and be able to realize and act on his or her full potential, rather than being constrained by fear.

The person-centered therapist promotes trust by providing unflagging appreciation of the experience of the patient. This is carried out by the therapist's listening reflectively and trusting the perceptions and self-directive capacities of the clients. The client is expected to talk in therapy about whatever comes to mind.

A similar type of talk therapy is that of Rollo May's existential psychotherapy. What brings a person into therapy is assumed to be his or her underlying concerns about death, freedom, isolation from others, and the meaning of his life.

The existential therapist assists the patient to focus on how he avoids taking responsibility for his actions and feelings and to own his actions and feelings. Therapy techniques might include enactment of feelings or thoughts, participation in guided fantasy, or use of body techniques.

Although having its primary application in individual therapy, both humanistic and existential themes and insights have been applied extensively in group therapy. In groups, patients learn how their behavior is viewed by others, how it makes others feel and influences their opinions, and how all of this ultimately influences the patient's opinion of herself.

The duration of therapy using a humanistic/existential approach varies. Individual therapy may last months or years. A group experience may span a single weekend or convene weekly for a fixed period of time or on an ongoing basis.

Family Systems

The family systems approach to therapy is relatively new on the therapy scene. The "patient" is the entire family or the couple. A central concept is "circularity," by which is meant that pathology or dysfunction is not caused by one person or by events in the past but by the ongoing, circular interactions of the participants, including the therapist.

An important concept for understanding human interactions is that of the "triangle." When two people come into conflict in a family, a third person—usually another family member—is often "triangulated" into the interaction. One aim of family therapy may be to de-triangulate the interaction and to promote the family members to deal more directly and constructively with the conflict.

The therapist may use a variety of different techniques in family system therapy, including assigning homework, reframing the way the family members understand the problem, or helping the members of the system to develop a "genogram"—a kind of emotional family tree or diagram of relationships within the family.

Family therapy sessions usually last about an hour and a half, and are often spaced several weeks apart. Therapy ends when the family members are better able to manage the problem they came in to therapy to fix. This usually takes between one and 20 sessions.

Therapist Titles and Credentials

Therapists have different kinds of training leading to various academic or professional degrees. There are four so-called "core providers" of mental health services: psychiatrists, clinical psychologists, psychiatric social workers, and psychiatric nurses.[3] Additional care providers include counselors of various types and therapists-in-training.

Psychiatrist

Psychiatry is the medical specialty that seeks to study, diagnose, and treat "mental illness." A psychiatrist holds a degree from a medical school (generally an M.D.), and has generally completed a three or four year residency focusing on mental health/mental illness problems. Psychiatrists are uniquely qualified to prescribe psychotropic medications (antidepressants, antipsychotics, etc.), as well as to prescribe and administer special treatments such as electroconvulsive shock treatment.

Some psychiatrists (as well as other care providers) become psychoanalysts. To do so, he or she must undergo several additional years of specialized training and supervision provided by a psychoanalytic institute, as well as participate in his own personal psychoanalysis, to be qualified to represent himself as a psychoanalyst.

Not all physicians who practice psychiatry have necessarily undergone any special training or passed the medical specialty board in psychiatry. In the United States, any physician licensed to practice medicine can choose to practice treatment of a particular type of illness, including mental illness. Thus, a physician with just an internship in general medicine may hang out a shingle stating he practices psychiatry. It is important to check credentials. Generally, board-certified psychiatrists are more likely to possess the greatest knowledge of the field.

Clinical Psychologist

Psychologists providing mental health services may hold either a Ph.D. or a Psy.D. degree. In addition to completing a formal internship, they receive training in one or more of the major therapeutic orientations mentioned above, and may specialize in a particular area of psychology. Clinical psychologists are specifically trained in psychodiagnostic testing and clinical research. They do not prescribe medications.

Almost all states now require a Ph.D. or Psy.D. for licensure or registration as a clinical psychologist and to maintain an independent practice. However, not all licensed Ph.D. psychologists practicing clinical psychology have extensive training in clinical practice. Much of a Ph.D.'s training is in statistics and research methodology, even though relatively few end up following a research career. (By contrast, the Psy.D. degree reflects emphasis on clinical training.)

Clinical psychologists may work in hospitals, mental health clinics, or private practice. Some teach and do research. Again, inquire into credentials and training.

Psychiatric Social Worker

In order to become a psychiatric social worker, it is necessary to complete a two-year master's degree program in social work leading to a M.S.W. degree and to get specialized training in psychiatry. The psychiatric social worker gets special training in either casework (providing social services and counseling to individuals and families with medical, legal, economic, or social problems), group work (working with youth groups, senior citizen groups, minority groups, etc.), or community organization (working with civic, religious, political, or industrial groups to develop community-wide programs to address particular problems).

In the course of their work, psychiatric social workers engage in verbal psychotherapy with clients experiencing problems of living. Their unique expertise is their knowledge and utilization of the community welfare resources available to the client and the client's family.

Psychiatric Nurse

In addition to being a registered nurse (R.N.), a psychiatric nurse possesses a master's degree and specialized training in the care of mental patients. Although most psychiatric nurses work in mental hospitals or clinics, some are in private practice, in which case they are more involved in supervising treatment regimens and individual therapy.

Psychoanalyst

A psychoanalyst is generally a psychiatrist, psychologist, or social worker, who has received specialized training from a psychoanalytic institute. A psychoanalyst has also completed his or her own psychoanalysis as part of the training.

Counselor

Counselor is a generic term that designates a person who holds a master's (M.A.) or a doctorate (Ph.D., Ed.D., Psy.D.) from an accredited graduate school program in clinical or counseling psychology, and who has completed a supervised internship. Types of counselors include school counselors, career counselors, rehabilitation counselors, correctional counselors, addiction counselors, and employment counselors.

Marriage, Family, and Child Counselor

A marriage and family therapist is specially trained in working with the family as a unit and resolving marital or family discord. He or she possesses either a master's or a doctoral degree and is certified by the American Association for Marriage and Family Therapy. An MFCC also completes an internship. Generally, MFCCs charge less than either psychiatrists or clinical psychologists for psychotherapy.

Pastoral Counselor

A pastoral counselor holds a degree from a theological school and a master's or doctorate in pastoral counseling or a related mental health discipline. Certification by the American Association of Pastoral Counselors requires experience in ministry and extensive supervision and practice in counseling and psychotherapy. Not all clergy are trained to provide mental health counseling, although most are trained to recognize serious emotional problems and to make referrals for outside help when necessary.

Therapists-in-Training and Psychological Assistants

Low fee clinics and programs, as well as a number of government-support agencies such as county mental health programs, use therapists-in-training to provide services to their patients or clients. These are people who are currently enrolled in a program of graduate study, usually in clinical or counseling psychology, and who are completing requirements for their internship. They are not paid for their services.

Once a therapist-in-training has been awarded a master's or a doctoral degree, but has not yet passed the licensing exam, he or she may apply to be a psychological assistant and may apprentice herself to a licensed care provider such as a licensed clinical psychologist. Generally a psychological assistant can provide high quality therapy at a low fee.

Other Mental Health Professionals

Volunteer crisis hotline workers tend to have less traditional training. Their knowledge of psychotherapy and crisis intervention usually comes from first-hand experience and in-service training.

Choosing a Therapist

When choosing a therapist, you need to consider not only the prospective therapist's credentials, but also your needs and reactions to him or her.

Psychotherapy is most effective when you feel relatively comfortable with your therapist. Feelings of trust are especially important. You don't need to agree with your therapist on every issue, but on large issues, especially issues that are important to you, you and your therapist should be in agreement.

If you are an incest survivor, you may want to work with a therapist who has training or experience in this area. If you are gay or lesbian, you may prefer a therapist of similar persuasion. If your issues center around problems with people of the opposite sex, you may feel more comfortable working with a same sex therapist.

The First Contact

Don't be afraid to interview several potential therapists before committing to one. Take into account your impressions at the first contact—which is likely to be prior to your first face-to-face meeting. Your first contact may well be by the telephone or telephone answering machine—you may need to leave a message for the therapist to get back to you.

Some important impressions to filter into your decision include: Was the message on the machine brief and professional? Did the therapist return your call promptly—within hours or a day or two at the most?

What to Watch For

When you first make contact with a prospective therapist, indicate your wish for a consultation and indicate who referred you. Note whether the therapist was friendly but professional on the phone.

The therapist should be able to give you relevant information on the phone to set up the appointment—he should inquire about the urgency of your situation, establish a time, give directions, respond to questions about fee—without engaging in extraneous comments, such as telling you about himself, where he went to school, or what he believes about therapeutic technique. Did you get the impression your call was handled while someone else was in the therapist's office, or did your conversation suggest privacy and confidentiality? During your first contact, did your interaction with the therapist convey a sense of his or her concern and warmth, or was it cold and perfunctory?

Urgency

Be sure to make clear to the therapist at your first contact whether you experiencing any severe symptoms—feeling suicidal, deeply depressed, uncontrollably angry—or whether there has been some acute crisis—a sudden death of a loved one, an upsetting medical diagnosis, etc. If the therapist seems to ignore symptoms or disregard the importance to you of these issues, or if he or she cannot give you an appointment within a few days, seek another, more available and responsive therapist.

Establishing a Fee

If you, as a prospective patient, can afford to pay no more than a certain amount, discuss this with the therapist, preferably at the first contact. Most therapists are willing to work with you to establish a fee you can afford, or they can make a referral to a therapist who can accommodate your ability to pay.

Self-Prescribing

Sometimes patients have definite ideas about the kinds of interventions or techniques they feel would help solve their problem. For example, some people want hypnosis as a short-cut to getting rid of certain health habits, such as overeating or smoking, or to uncover "the real problem."

Generally, patients should not prescribe their own treatment. Hypnosis and similar interventions may or may not be an appropriate part of a larger treatment plan, but the therapist is in the best position to determine this. Most certainly it is appropriate to discuss your ideas with your therapist; just be guided by his or her suggestions about the overall treatment approach.

Person-to-Person Considerations

When you first meet one-on-one with your therapist, some things to keep in mind are: Is his or her office maintained at his living quarters? If so, are you aware of, or do you run into, any members of his family when coming to the office? Does the therapist's office lack adequate soundproofing—can you hear what's being said in the therapist's office while you are waiting outside? If the answer is "yes" to these questions, you may want to reconsider your choice of a therapist.

Once you have begun working with a therapist, you should feel free to raise questions and share difficult feelings, even if they are directed at the therapist. It is okay to be angry with a therapist—as long as you let him or her know. You should expect your therapist to listen and be concerned, to ask for clarification when necessary, and to avoid revealing much about himself or herself that is of a personal nature. Most therapists avoid being physically demonstrative—hugging or touching their patients with anything more than a reassuring pat when appropriate. Sexual contact by a therapist is *never* a legitimate aspect of therapy.

If your therapist talks too much, constantly interrupts you to ask questions, talks about himself or herself a lot, falls asleep in session, is usually late or doesn't end on time, takes phone calls during your session, repeatedly changes the time and/or day of the sessions, or otherwise acts unprofessionally, consider changing therapists.

If your therapist comes on to you sexually, is verbally abusive or physically assaultive, offers to exchange therapy for your services, or suggests terminating your therapy relationship in order to have a personal one, you should immediately stop seeing him or her and talk to a different therapist about this situation.

Termination

How long therapy should last is often a concern for both patients and therapists. Except for behavior therapy and certain time-limited approaches, most therapy is open ended. Usually therapy ends when symptoms are alleviated or when the patient's ability to cope with problems improves significantly. If you and your therapist have established specific goals for therapy, you and the therapist may choose to end therapy when these have been attained or when you feel substantial and adequate progress toward these goals has been made.

It is reasonable to ask your therapist how you and she will know when therapy should terminate and how it will be handled. Often it is the patient who introduces the possibility of ending therapy. When this happens, you and she will usually set a date for termination about four to six weeks hence. In some cases, therapy may end prematurely, as when the therapist must move to a different internship or clinic. If you are not ready to end therapy altogether, your therapist should arrange for a timely transfer of your case to another therapist.

It is normal, when the time comes to terminate, for the patient to feel sad or even upset about this change. These feelings, and the gains made as well as the shortfalls of therapy, need to be discussed prior to termination.

Group Therapy

Occasionally patients who are being seen individually by a therapist also participate in group psychotherapy. When one participates in individual and group therapy sessions concurrently, it is called "combined therapy." The idea is that the group experience should interact meaningfully with the individual therapy experience.

As with individual therapy, there are many different approaches to group therapy. Clinicians with a psychoanalytic frame of reference will focus the group's attention on how patterns of interacting between group members and the therapist actually repeat old patterns from childhood. By contrast, a transactional therapy group will emphasize the "here-and-now" games people play with each other.

A behavioral group will learn to analyze dysfunctional behavior patterns and to provide the right environment and reinforcement for new patterns to emerge and take hold. A gestalt group will enable participants to get in touch with feelings and express them openly and honestly. A psychodrama group will stage a dramatization of an emotion-laden situation to help its members gain insight. No matter what the theoretical orientation or techniques employed, an important factors in all group therapy is that participants come to realize that they are not alone in having a problem, that others may be struggling with the same or similar problems. The simple sharing of experiences fills an important human need.

Self-Help Groups

Increasingly, self-help groups are a means of meeting members' needs to share problems by providing acceptance, mutual support, and help. Self-help groups run the gamut from informal independent gatherings to complex national and even international organizations with hundreds of local chapters and thousands of members.

Most groups are organized around a particular issue or problem, such as alcohol abuse or incest. They do not attempt to explore individual psychodynamics in great depth or to change personality functioning significantly. Nevertheless, self-help groups have improved the emotional health and well-being of many people.

The help such groups offer is direct, concrete, and empathic. The crucial component is immediate, wordless identification. There is no need to give a lengthy explanation of the problem. The other group members already know from personal experience what you have experienced and are feeling. Not only does a group member feel understood and accepted, she has the opportunity to work through her related feelings and difficulties by being able to reach out and help others cope with a similar problem.

Although some self-help groups are founded by professionals, they tend to be steered by group members themselves, sometimes with trained specialists serving as consultants. Furthermore, physicians and mental health professionals routinely refer their clients to self-help groups.

Despite the advocacy for self-help and the support provided by professionals, some self-help group members spurn formal therapy. This is especially true for people who have been in self-help groups a long time and remember the days when professional therapists and self-help groups were at odds. In other cases, people who have had bad experiences with therapists but who have found support in a self-help group may reject the possibility that formal therapy can be helpful as well.

Hazards of Self-Help Groups

Despite the overwhelming positive aspects of self-help groups, the potential for harm exists. Some groups are so committed to the idea of self-revelation that they may push a new member to reveal too much too fast. When this happens, the person may flee the group, feeling naked and vulnerable for having "told all." In the worst possible case, the person could have a serious mental breakdown.

Another hazard of some self-help groups is over-diagnosing themselves with popular labels gleaned from the psychiatric profession or from the media. Thus, some people who join an incest survivors self-help group are told, "If you are an incest survivor, you must have multiple personalities." Such a pronouncement can be overwhelming to the new member, who is already having difficulty coping with the aftermath of incest. In fact, the diagnosis of Multiple Personality Disorder is very difficult to make for even the best-trained professionals.

Still another problem occurs when a group member needs acceptance and support but gets rejected. This can occur when the member is trying to find a sponsor, or when she does not comply with the sponsor's rules. In one instance, a man who was schizophrenic could not get another person to be his sponsor in a 12-step program, despite his ability to function well in society. Another woman's sponsor refused to continue with her after she ended up in a psychiatric hospital and was prescribed medications for her illness. Still another person was rejected by her sponsor because she wished to get into individual therapy as well as be in a 12-step program.

Those who go to self-help groups are not necessarily screened. Thus, the groups attract individuals with a wide range of problems, including people with severe mental disorders. Such people can induce alarm in other group members, especially if they become emotionally unstable or begin to dominate the group. Without the intervention of a person trained to handle such problems, it is easy for a group member to feel overwhelmed by another's problems.

These occasional abuses aside, however, most self-help groups regard themselves as a complement to, rather than a replacement for therapy or medical treatment, and they don't discourage members from seeking other assistance.

Self-Help vs. Scam

Even though most self-help groups are legitimate, you need to take responsibility for protecting yourself by shopping wisely for self-help. There are people using the mantle of self-help to further their own schemes.

Sometimes a self-help group is nothing more than a guise for attracting clients to individual counseling sessions with someone who may or may not be professionally trained to provide services. In other cases, the group is a publicity vehicle for the authors of pop-psychology books.

If the group charges more than $5 per meeting, or doesn't have face-to-face meetings, or isn't self-determining—beware; it may not be self-help. If you attend a self-help group and its members attempt to diagnose you, or if you feel upset or alarmed at their behavior or actions, do not be afraid to refuse any further contact with them. Check out the group beforehand if possible, to determine their legitimacy.

Information on Self-Help Groups

The ascendancy of the self-help movement, and its endorsement by the President's Commission on Mental Health, has led to the establishment of a number of regional self-help clearinghouses throughout the country. Each clearinghouse collects and disseminates information about local self-help groups and helps people organize new ones. They also provide training to both lay people and professionals, sponsor research, publish directories of local self-help groups, and function as referral networks.

Appendix A lists the self-help clearinghouses throughout the country that you can contact for further information on an issue of interest to you. *Appendix B* gives a partial list of resource organizations, listed by focus, that can serve as a starting place for locating help near you.

Reaching Out for Weight Management Help

When food and eating is used to suppress feelings related to old wounds such as sexual or physical abuse, or when it is a means of distracting attention from present-day sources of emotional pain, such as the loss of a job or a loved one, additional help may be needed to keep the pounds from returning. Seeking therapy from a qualified professional or joining an appropriate self-help group may provide the needed assistance.

Continuing in the maintenance program of your weight control program, or getting additional weight management support is also important. This is one of the strategies that characterizes those who have attained long-lasting weight control success. One criterion for selecting a weight loss program is whether it provides adequate and long-term support for maintenance as well as for weight loss.

Another alternative is to employ the services of a registered dietitian (R.D.) to provide you with additional dietary counseling and weight management support. Although usually employed in hospitals and community agencies, more and more dietitians are going into private practice or conducting their own weight control programs. Dietitians are especially good at teaching innovative ways of managing food, and they are specially trained to translate nutrition requirements into healthful, tasty diets.

However, beware of impostors. Because the titles "nutritionist" and "nutrition consultant" are unregulated in most states, any one, even those without recognized credentials, can adopt this label. In addition, a small number of licensed professionals are engaged in unscientific nutrition practices.

Summary

Reaching out for help may mean getting psychotherapy, particularly if there are difficult issues that you have been unable to resolve on your own, or when eating has been used to deal with painful emotions associated with past trauma. Another avenue of assistance is to join a relevant self-help group.

In addition to exercising and controlling calories, continuing to get support for weight management after having reached goal weight is a key factor in long-term success. This may involve participating in a formal maintenance program that is an extension of your weight loss program, enrolling in a further weight-loss program, or using the services of a dietitian.

Being willing to reach out for additional help will increase your chances for long-term weight management success.

References

1.   Langs, R., (1989). *Rating Your Psychotherapist*. New York: Ballantine Books..

2.   Frank, J.D. (1985). Therapeutic components shared by all psychotherapies. In M.J. Mahoney and A. Freeman (Eds.), *Cognition and Psychotherapy*. NY: Plenum Press. (pp. 49–70)

3.   Hershenson, D.B., & Power, P.W. (1987). *Mental Health Counseling: Theory and Practice*. NY: Pergamon Press.

Chapter 12

Coping With Success

JOHN HAD LOST 32 pounds and had 8 to go to reach his goal weight of 180. He had also lost his beer belly and extra chin, and he was feeling wonderful about his accomplishments. But he complained that friends who on the one hand told him how good he looked, also cautioned him not to lose too much more weight, and even expressed alarm about his present health.

"As a young adult I weighed 180, and that's within the range suggested in the desirable height and weight tables for a man my height, but now I'm not sure. How do I know when I've really reached a good weight for me, and once I do, how do I eat so that I stay at that weight?"

Norma had lost 45 pounds, and even though she still had 25 to go to reach goal weight, she noticed that several of the men at work were starting to linger around her desk. She loved the compliments she was getting from everyone about how terrific she looked; but at the same time, the attention made her nervous. She wasn't sure what others really expected of her, and she was beginning to worry about the last 25 pounds.

Maggie's parents contributed the money for her to go to a prestigious live-in weight reduction program. She knew they were doing it because they wanted her to be happier, and they thought losing weight would help. When she returned from the center, she had reached her goal weight, but she still felt depressed. Even though she had lost weight, life wasn't any better, and now she felt she had disappointed her parents and misspent their money.

John, Norma, and Maggie's stories are just three examples of the difficulty of coping with successful weight loss. While people in the early stages of the weight losing battle may feel "I wish I had that problem," reaching goal weight brings with it a whole new set of problems that can be just as difficult as those faced trying to get there. The first difficulty comes in deciding when you have in fact reached a goal weight with which you can live.

Finalizing Your Maintenance Goal Weight

Deciding when to stop losing weight and switch to maintaining goal weight isn't as easy as it may seem. You may disagree with what the height-weight tables recommend, or with what the doctor or nutritionist says. If you have never been "normal" weight, or haven't been slim for quite some time, you may have no idea what you should "ideally" weigh. Using some historical criterion, such as deciding you want to weigh what you weighed in high school, may not be realistic for your current lifestyle—or the adult body you now have.

Some people argue that you should aim to maintain a weight at which you "feel best." The problem is, such a subjective weight goal doesn't clearly define a goal, and it is too easy when temptation presents itself to convince yourself that you could "feel better" at a higher (or lower) weight. Uncertainty about what you should weigh can destabilize your weight management success in the long-run. You need to have a definite idea about the best weight for you.

Two questions need to be answered for you to decide what weight is really "best" for you:

1. What is a healthy weight for me?

2. What weight am I willing to live with?

What Is a "Healthy" Weight?

Determining your best or most healthy weight isn't easy. The most common means of assessing body weight is to refer to some height-weight table. A variety of such tables exist, which give ranges of "ideal" weights adjusted for sex and sometimes for other variables, such as frame size.

All have been seriously criticized for a number of reasons: the methodology used to obtain the data for constructing the table introduces bias; important variables such as age and frame size are not incorporated into the table in a meaningful way; the recommended weight ranges are arbitrary; even the concept that there is such a thing as an "ideal" body weight that can be defined for a given person is being challenged by some experts.

It is certainly true that a person whose weight is at the outer edge of the weight distribution—who is either very fat or very thin—has a much greater health risk. It is less certain at what point a person whose weight falls in the mid-range is at a higher health risk.

Current research suggests that health risk is relatively low over a wide range of weights between the extremes of underweight and obesity. How much health risk you are subject to depends largely on your age. Younger people—those under 20 or 25—are at much greater risk for developing health problems when they have even small amounts of excess weight. By contrast, the older a person gets, the more excess weight he or she can carry and still not incur much additional health risk.

Other variables besides age influence health risk from higher weights. If you have a family history of hypertension, heart disease, hypercholesterolemia, cancer, or diabetes, you would be wiser to maintain a lower body weight.

Similarly, determining when weight is too low for good health is a problem, albeit a somewhat easier one. A few health gurus advocate maintaining body weight at a level substantially below normal weight as defined by height-weight table ranges. However, a body weight 15% or more below average weight for women or 25% below for men, depending on age, is generally recognized as a significant health hazard.

So how can you decide what is a healthy weight for you—a weight you should attempt to maintain? You should consider several pieces of data in making this decision.

Despite the problems inherent in height-weight tables, this is one place to begin. Look at Table 12.1 and find the weight range for your height and sex. (Disregard the frame size designations—these are only arbitrary, and most people don't have any way of knowing what their frame size is.)

If you are a young person, especially if you are under age 25, focus on the *lower* end of the recommended range, or use the range for "small" frame size if it is given. If you are older, you may be better off to use the *upper* limits. If you are over 50, the "large" frame size range may be more appropriate because it gives a relatively higher range.

Other data you may wish to obtain and use in your deliberation on what a healthy weight might be for you might include a body composition analysis, your Body Mass Index, and your waist-to-hips ratio.

Body Composition Analysis

Whether a given weight is healthy really depends on the proportion of fat to lean body mass. Some people have a relatively high body weight but a low percentage of fat, while others may be within or even below their "desirable" range according to the height and weight tables, but still be quite fat.[1] It is impossible to tell if you are at a healthy body weight by using just a weight scale, because the important criterion is not body weight but body composition.

Ideally, men should carry 15% or less of their body weight in fat. The recommended desirable level for women is generally given as 20%, although some experts go as high as 25%. The acceptable level of body fat rises with age, but it is generally agreed that a man is too fat if more than 20% of his body weight is from fat. A woman is too fat if more than 30% of her body weight is fat.

Table 12.1

*1983 Metropolitan Height & Weight Table**

Weights are for ages 25–59 based on lowest mortality. Weights include indoor clothing weight 3 lbs. for women and 5 lbs. for men. Heights include shoes with 1" heels.

Height	Small Frame	Medium Frame	Large Frame
Men			
5' 2"	128–134	131–141	138–150
5' 3"	130–136	133–143	140–153
5' 4"	132–138	135–145	142–156
5' 5"	134–140	137–148	144–160
5' 6"	136–142	139–151	146–164
5' 7"	138–145	142–154	149–168
5' 8"	140–148	145–157	152–172
5' 9"	142–151	148–160	155–176
5'10"	144–154	151–163	158–180
5'11"	146–157	154–166	161–184
6'	149–160	157–170	164–188
6' 1"	152–164	160–174	168–192
6' 2"	155–168	164–178	172–197
6' 3"	158–172	167–182	176–202
6' 4"	162–176	171–187	181–207
Women			
4'10"	102–111	109–121	118–131
4'11"	103–113	111–123	120–134
5'	104–115	113–126	122–137
5' 1"	106–118	115–129	125–140
5' 2"	108–121	118–132	128–143
5' 3"	111–124	121–135	131–147
5' 4"	114–127	124–138	134–151
5' 5"	117–130	127–141	137–155
5' 6"	120–133	130–144	140–159
5' 7"	123–136	133–147	143–163
5' 8"	126–139	136–150	146–167
5' 9"	129–142	139–153	149–170
5'10"	132–145	142–156	152–173
5'11"	135–148	145–159	155–176
6'	138–151	148–162	158–179

*Courtesy of Metropolitan Life Insurance Company

If you have been involved in a program of regular aerobic exercise, you are likely to have added muscle mass to your body at the same time you have reduced fat stores. This will affect your fat to lean body ratio, and make it possible for you to weigh more but at the same time be less fat! Therefore, you may need to revise your maintenance goal weight upwards if your body composition analysis shows that you are at a healthy ratio of fat to lean body mass. After all, it is not what you weigh that counts but how fat you are.

Serious athletes tend to have very low levels of fat. World class male marathon runners have been found to have between 4% and 8% body fat. Women athletes frequently fall in the range of 8% to 13%. The leanest woman distance runner was assessed at 5.9% fat, while some pro-football defensive backs have measured as low as 1% body fat.

A certain amount of body fat is needed for good health. It is generally believed that less than 4% fat in males or 10% fat in females may prove dangerous. When body fat is too low, women may stop having menstrual periods and have difficulty getting pregnant.

The most accurate method for determining body composition is by *hydrostatic* or *underwater weighing*. This involves getting into a large tub of water, sitting on a seat connected to a scale, and ducking your head under water long enough to be weighed. For people who are frightened of water, this can be intimidating.

An alternative to weighing under water is to have body composition determined through *skinfold* (actually "fatfold") *measurement*. This is done by a trained technician using skinfold calipers and taking measurements at various sites on the body. Unfortunately, unless the measurement is taken by an experienced technician with high-quality calipers, a number of things can go wrong, leading to an inaccurate reading.

A number of health clubs are now offering a *computerized body composition assessment* using electrodes that are attached to the skin. Although this high-tech approach would seem to be a fool-proof method of getting an accurate reading, it often is not.

In fact, with all three methods the underlying formulae and data base used to calculate body composition introduce bias. The data were developed from studies with young, white males, and are not likely to be directly applicable to other groups.

Given that all of these methods are prone to error, the best approach is to get several "readings," preferably using more than one method. Then, you should regard each of these as additional data points to take into consideration in determining the best body weight for you. You may wish to take an average of the various data points, or just arbitrarily choose the range that feels right, given all the data you have gathered, and considering your age and your family health history.

Unfortunately, it is not possible to give an average or healthy weight

Table 12.2

Height Converted to Meters

(Denominator for BMI Formula)

Height in Inches	Height in Meters Squared (Height²)	Height in Inches	Height in Meters Squared (Height²)
56	2.01	67	2.89
57	2.10	68	2.99
58	2.16	69	3.06
59	2.25	70	3.17
60	2.31	71	3.24
61	2.40	72	3.35
62	2.46	73	3.42
63	2.56	74	3.53
64	2.66	75	3.61
65	2.72	76	3.72
66	2.82	77	3.83

*Courtesy of Metropolitan Life Insurance Company

range that applies to everyone. Just remember—lower is usually better, up to a point, as long as you don't start obsessing about your weight or worrying so much that your ability to enjoy life is compromised. The older you are, the more latitude you have.

Body Mass Index

Another measure of fatness that correlates highly with more direct measures of body fat is the *Body Mass Index*. Typically this is calculated by dividing weight in kilograms by height in meters squared (W/H²).

Some experts have argued that the W/H² formula doesn't take into account the naturally higher proportion of body fat that women have versus men. To try and account for this, researchers use different cutpoints for men and women.

Using this formula, a "desirable" *Body Mass Index* for men is generally assumed to be 22 to 24, and for women 21 to 23. Health risk is believed to be elevated above 28.5 for men and 27.5 for women. Above 33 for men and 31.5 for women indicates seriously increased health risk. Again, higher scores are acceptable with increasing age.

To calculate your *Body Mass Index*, first, convert your body weight in pounds to kilograms by dividing weight in pounds by 2.205. The result you obtain is the numerator (number above the line) in the BMI formula.

Formula to Convert Weight in lbs. to kg.

Your weight: _____ = _____
Divided by: 2.205   (weight in kg.)

To get the denominator (number below the line) for the BMI formula, look up your height in inches on the table on the preceding page, and then find the correct height in meters squared.

Now that you have the numerator (weight in kilograms) and the denominator (height in meters squared), you can proceed to calculate the formula to determine your *Body Mass Index.*

Formula for Calculating Body Mass Index

Divide body weight in kilograms by height in meters squared.

$$BMI = \frac{\text{Weight (in kg)}}{\text{Height}^2 \text{ (in meters)}} =$$

Waist-to-Hips Ratio

Another piece of data that may be useful for judging healthy weight is the waist-to-hips ratio. *Where* fat is deposited is an important predictor of whether overweight is a health hazard. Fat in the waist, flank, and abdomen is more metabolically active, and more likely to be associated with diabetes, hypertension, elevated lipid levels, stroke, coronary heart disease, and overall increased mortality, than fat in the thighs and buttocks. The higher the ratio of your waist measurement to hip measurement, the greater the risk.

You can find your ratio simply by measuring your waist and hips, and dividing the waist measurement by the hip measurement. If you are a man and have a ratio of 1.0 or less or if you are a woman and have a ratio of 0.8 or less, your weight distribution does not suggest elevated risk.

What Weight Can You Live With?

Health is just one criterion to use in choosing a maintenance goal weight. As you get older, and if you have a relatively risk-free family history, you can probably weigh more than some people would consider "ideal" and yet still be healthy. It is important that you choose a maintenance goal weight that you can live with and maintain—not one that someone else thinks is right or that society holds up as the standard of beauty.

In choosing a maintenance goal weight, you must seek the balance between the effort required to maintain a particular weight and how acceptable that goal weight is to you. Some people are not willing to spend the time and energy nor make the sacrifices required to reach and hold a lower goal weight. They are willing to accept a higher goal weight for the trade-off of not having to work too hard to maintain it.

One woman decided to settle on 145 as her maintenance weight, even though she felt she could reach 130 or 135 (which she had weighed at a younger age), if she put her mind to it. "My husband and I entertain a lot and I'm just not willing to make the sacrifices I would have to make in order to do that. I exercise and watch what I eat, but my life isn't devoted to exercising and minimizing calories. Ideally, I'd like to be 130 again, but I can live with 145 and be happy."

Still other people may feel they must maintain a really low weight to be able to look themselves in the mirror each day. They are willing to spend hours a day at the gym and do what it takes to stay at a lower goal weight. As long as this does not produce a binge-purge cycle or impair job or social functioning, and the weight sought meets the criterion for being healthy, this is probably okay.

The cross-over point, at which you may be physically able to lose more weight, but you aren't willing to make the effort, is the weight you are willing to live with. It is the weight that supports your psychological health. If this point also provides for your physical health, it is perfectly acceptable, in fact preferable to choose to maintain at this level—even though it may not match society's ideal for thinness.

Be careful, however, that the weight you are willing to live with is in the healthy zone; that is, it is neither too high nor too low. If it is too high, you are probably underrating your ability to achieve a healthy weight, or you have decided that since you can't achieve society's ideal of thinness, you may as well not bother at all. If it is too low, you may be in the clutches of an eating disorder, and you should seek professional help.

Once you decide to maintain a goal weight that is healthy, both physically and psychologically, even if it is higher than "ideal," stop worrying about losing more weight. Accept your decision, maintain this weight, and focus on enjoying your life. Don't let the next pencil-thin woman you meet throw you into a mental comparison between yourself and her to the point that you decide you are not okay and must go on another diet.

Periodically fretting about the discrepancy between what you have chosen to weigh and some unrealistic standard that you may or may not be able to attain will merely increase your anxiety level, make you more susceptible to quickie weight loss schemes, and possibly trigger emotional eating and consequent weight gain. Once you finalize a maintenance goal weight that is healthy and acceptable to you, the challenge is to maintain it.

Overcoming Factors That Undermine Success

It might seem that reaching your maintenance goal weight would be reward enough to maintain success. Yet many, if not most people who achieve weight loss success will attest to the difficulties involved in maintaining it. Life is not always better or easier thinner. The person at goal weight is not always happier and doesn't necessarily feel better about herself. There are often new terrors to confront and stresses to cope with from unexpected sources. The factors that undermine success are many.

Just what biochemical or physiological factors may be involved in regaining weight are not yet known. Some of the psychological factors that can undermine success in maintaining goal weight include:

... having difficulty handling compliments and expectations,

... still seeing yourself as an overweight person,

... not feeling worthy and not believing in yourself,

... obsessing about regaining weight,

... getting overconfident,

... having few other sources of rewards in life,

... focusing on weight rather than the real problem,

... having unreasonable expectations for what weight loss can do, and

... struggling for control over food and eating.

Difficulty Handling Compliments and Expectations

When Norma weighed 210 pounds, it was simply "business as usual" with her coworkers. By the time she had reached 165 pounds on her way to 140, however, things had changed. With all the compliments and unaccustomed attention, she wasn't sure how to act.

At first she just smiled and thanked people for their comments, sometimes sharing some part of her story of how she had achieved her weight management success. Eventually, however, she began to worry about letting others down if she didn't succeed in losing another 25 pounds.

What would they say if she regained the weight? She felt as if her eating was under constant surveillance, and she began to long for some relief from the constant tension of living up to others' expectations. By comparison, weighing 210 pounds had been like being invisible.

To make matters worse, Norma already had a boyfriend and didn't want to jeopardize that relationship, yet she was flattered and intrigued by the possibility of a new relationship with one of the men in the office. And now her present boyfriend had begun to complain that she was too thin and should gain some weight.

Norma's role in the office, and the implicit rules that govern all relationships, had changed along with her weight. The difficulty arose because she did not realize that that was likely to happen, and she was not sure in what way her role or the rules had changed. She was unsure of what others expected of her, and she had to confront her own fear of success.

Learning how to handle compliments and adjusting to changed expectations of others is a common hazard of success, but a challenge you must master. First, be sure that when someone is giving you a compliment you are not mentally discounting what they are saying, thinking catastrophizing or self-sabotaging thoughts such as, "What if I don't get to goal weight?" Make sure you avoid responding with a self put-down such as, "Well, I didn't have a good week this week."

Thinking traps that produce negative self-talk can turn well-meant compliments into mental poison. Learn to accept compliments as rightfully deserved, and use them to reaffirm to yourself your self-worth. Use your imagination and mentally practice receiving compliments, taking them in a positive way, and responding appropriately.

When compliments no longer have a positive effect, speak up for what you really want. Start by thanking the person offering the compliment, and then tell them how it is affecting you and what you would prefer they do. "You are so wonderful to notice my weight loss, and I know it sounds crazy, but I'm starting to feel pressured by all the attention I'm getting. What I'd most like right now is just to be treated like everyone else, so could you please not compliment me so much. Perhaps you could save it all up, and in a few months when I get to my permanent goal weight, then give me a card or something with a few compliments. Thanks so much for your understanding."

Changed expectations present another sort of hazard. At 210 pounds, Norma knew what was expected of her and how to act. At 165 she wasn't sure whether the attention she was getting from men in the office indicated a romantic interest or curiosity. At first her boyfriend had been quite positive about her weight loss, but now he seemed to want something else from her.

Although you will always be influenced to some degree by others' expectations for how you should be and act, it is important to sort out what you want for yourself versus what others want for you. If you doubt your own self-worth, you may tend to place too much emphasis on what others expect of you, but if you can clarify and keep in mind those values you hold dear, you are likely to be guided by your own values and expectations. This means being willing to risk others' wrath if you refuse to conform to their point of view.

Norma had to first decide for herself what she wanted—the excitement of a new relationship or the comfort and contentment of an old one. Then she had to manage her self-talk so that she could take a firm stand and assert what she decided she wanted.

She had to confront and challenge limiting beliefs about whether she had what it took to interest a new man. She had to recognize that compliments and changing expectations are a normal part of the change process she had undertaken with weight management, and to ensure long-term success, she had to learn how to deal with them effectively.

Lagging Body Image

As long as she could remember, Karen had been heavy. As a child she was the fattest kid in her classes and the butt of many jokes. In her early 20s she slimmed down to a size 16, met and married her husband, and regained weight until she was a size 20. Her mental picture of herself was that of a large woman.

When she joined a weight control program and began losing weight, her body image didn't keep up. Unexpected glimpses of her slimmer body in plate glass windows startled her. When she went shopping for clothes, she first went to the size she was used to buying. Discovering in the fitting room that the clothes were too large, she went to the next size down, which still turned out to be too large. Finally she would become so upset because she didn't know what size she took that she would leave the store without a purchase.

When others told her how slim she was, she wasn't sure whether they were speaking to her or to someone nearby. Once she realized the comment was directed to her, she wasn't sure whether it was really meant as a compliment.

Updating Your Body Image

Like Karen, you may have a hard time accepting the new, slimmer you. It may be helpful to use guided imagery to help your body image catch up with your weight loss success. In this way you practice seeing yourself slimmer and interacting with others as a slimmer person.

It helps to do this in stages, starting first with visualizing yourself ten or 20 pounds lighter than your present weight, and then moving to successively slimmer images. Mentally picture how your body looks both nude and wearing slimmer clothes. Mentally see yourself in social situations, and hear people giving you compliments. Practice thanking people for their remarks. Look them in the eye and allow yourself to accept what they say.

When you find yourself with old mental pictures of yourself, gently let go and bring to mind your new image, or go look in a mirror to remind yourself about the new you. Talk to yourself, and remind yourself that you worked hard for the New You, and you deserve it.

Issues With Self-Worth

Gwenn had lost 60 pounds. At 135 pounds, she looked really good, and her friends complimented her on her cute figure. Still, she was plagued with self-worth issues. Even though she was well educated and had held several responsible jobs in which she had done well before starting a new business venture with her husband, Gwenn doubted both her ability to create results, and also her ability to relate successfully to others.

Not believing in yourself may be the result of being frequently criticized by others, leading you to question your own self-worth. When you take unjust criticism to heart, you may even come to feel you don't deserve any better than you are getting. Such ideas are usually reinforced by sabotaging self-talk that further enmeshes you in a difficult situation and a context that works to undermine success.

To begin to overcome this factor, ask yourself where the self-deprecating notions come from. If you are caught in a difficult situation, what can you do to create a context that works to support success? If not believing in yourself comes from your own ideas of your abilities, and decisions you have made about yourself and what you deserve, you have to challenge these beliefs, and change your self-talk to be more accepting and supportive.

Try making a list of at least 20 "good news" things about yourself—your abilities, your good points, the things you like about yourself. If you have trouble generating 20 items, ask several friends (not the ones who are critical of you) to give you some suggestions derived from their experience with you. Then use this list to create supportive self-talk, and practice reminding yourself of these good qualities, especially when you are feeling down.

Fear of Regaining Weight

June had lost 65 pounds, and now maintained her weight primarily by teaching classes in weight management for a well-known weight loss organization. Even so, her days were filled with fear of regaining the weight. By dwelling on catastrophizing thoughts about how awful it would be to regain weight, she kept herself mesmerized by fear and distraught with anxiety.

To get herself out of her fear of regaining weight, June needed to use thought stopping when she found herself catastrophizing, and to refocus her thoughts to be supportive and self-assuring. She needed to remind herself that she had successfully lost 65 pounds, demonstrating that she had the ability to lose weight, and that she could always call on these skills when needed. She needed to focus her thoughts on fitness and on celebrating herself and her life, rather than on worrying about regaining weight. June also needed to learn techniques for overcoming and managing anxiety.

When you find yourself feeling afraid of regaining weight, you are looking backwards in your thoughts to all the effort and struggle it took to lose it. And you are letting yourself dwell on "how awful it would be" to gain it back.

You must get your thoughts turned around and focused on today and the future—your daily exercise goals, your long-term exercise challenge, making healthy food choices today, coping successfully today. Take it one step at a time, and don't get caught looking back too much; that could make your fears a reality.

Also, carefully review Chapter 7, *Overcoming Depression and Anxiety,* for suggestions for coping with anxiety.

Overconfidence

Just the opposite of fear of regaining weight, is overconfidence about maintaining. The essence of overconfidence is the thought that "I've got this knocked, and I don't have to worry about my weight any more." You may be drawn into overconfidence by the way your body responds to inappropriate eating once you are at goal weight.

If you have maintained goal weight for a while, you may discover that an occasional bout of inappropriate eating does not automatically cause a weight gain. It is as if you have a credit card with which you may charge excess calories without having to pay for them right away. This is because at lower weights, and especially if you are maintaining regular exercise, your body is more forgiving about excess calories—at least for a while.

After a series of excesses without commensurate weight gain, you may decide that you don't have to worry any more, that somehow you have become a naturally normal-weight person. This overconfidence may lead you to reduce or even abandon your exercise. Then suddenly, in a very short period of time—weeks or a month, you may experience rapid weight gain. Your credit for indulgences has run out, and you discover too late that you have a new weight problem.

Don't allow yourself to become overconfident. Be sure you have a means of monitoring your eating and your exercise habits, as well as your body weight. Keep tabs on yourself without becoming obsessive.

Managing weight effectively needs to be a lifetime hygiene habit, just like brushing your teeth. When you find yourself being tempted to be imprudent, remind yourself of the dangers of overconfidence. Don't kid yourself back into a weight problem.

Hooked on Losing

For some people, losing weight becomes very rewarding. They get a special pleasure out of stepping on the scale and hearing the balance beam go "thunk" as it indicates more pounds gone. This can insidiously become an "addiction," especially for those who have few other means of reward or pleasure in their lives. Once they reach goal weight, they may either keep on losing past the point of being healthy, or they may fall apart because they lose their only real source of reward.

To be successful once you reach goal weight, it is essential that you develop and internalize other ways to get pleasure than seeing the scale change. If you find yourself taking unusual pleasure in losing weight, examine what other sources of reward exist for you. Be sure you have completed the *20 Things I Love To Do* exercise on page 224, and review it. Begin immediately to build additional means of satisfaction into your life.

Overweight as a Solution

Sometimes being overweight is the solution, not the problem. Being overweight can be an excuse for not performing up to par, or not having to meet the expectations of others.

Zoe claimed that her weight had kept her from getting into an Ivy League school, and later from getting ahead in her job. Once she reached goal weight, she no longer had a good excuse for not doing her best and succeeding. Her fears that she could not really measure up, and her desire to thwart her mother's expectations for her led her to regain weight. Being overweight was the solution to her fears of failure, and her desire to get back at her mother.

Even though Zoe thought she wanted to be slimmer, she could not lose or maintain weight until she dealt with the real problem —her feelings about her mother and her mother's expectations. Until Zoe dealt with the real problem, her ability to maintain weight was minimal. Usually in cases such as Zoe's, the help of a mental health professional is required.

In addition to "solving" interpersonal issues, weight and weight control efforts can sometimes be the solution to boredom. Just as eating can be a solution to boredom because it gives you something to do, worrying about weight and attending a weight control program is also something to do. "Trying" to lose weight (or maintain it) but never quite succeeding fills up time and feels like something is being achieved, even if it isn't.

In some cases, a weight control group is the primary social network for a person. Reaching and maintaining goal weight usually redefines the person's status in the group as no longer "one of the gang" and reduces the opportunity for further socializing. Regaining weight can be a means of reinstituting connectedness—getting to be like your friends again. You may not even be aware that you are solving one problem by creating another.

If being at goal weight is uncomfortable for you, ask yourself if perhaps being overweight has served as a solution to some problem. If it has, you need to address the real problem, if you really want to maintain goal weight.

Unfulfilled Promises

Maggie hoped that by getting to goal weight she would finally feel better about herself, and find some satisfaction in life. But when she returned from the live-in weight reduction program her parents had sent her to, life was not better. She still didn't feel good about herself, and she knew it was just a matter of time before she regained the weight.

Getting to goal weight does not magically make life better. You are still likely to have the same old job, the same old relationships, and the same old problems. If, like Maggie, you hold onto the same old ways of thinking—being a perfectionist and constantly engaging in self-criticism—reaching goal weight may turn out to be an unfulfilled promise. Once you decide that "this isn't it and I'm not satisfied," regaining weight becomes a self-fulfilling prophecy, as you keep on seeking satisfaction in your life, usually through eating or drinking.

Be sure that the benefits you seek from weight reduction are realistic. If you are feeling unsatisfied even though you have reached goal weight, find the real reason why. Being at your goal weight cannot solve the real problems of your life—but to the extent that it is accompanied by a sense of accomplishment and elevated self-esteem, it can help you find and implement some solutions to your problems.

If the problem is a dead end job, being at goal weight can give you the confidence to seek a new job. If the problem is a relationship that takes from you more than it gives back, being at goal weight can give you the courage to seek a new relationship. If the problem is more illusive and undefined, being at goal weight can give you the strength to face and define the problem better, and that can point the way to an acceptable solution. Getting to goal weight can reduce your health risk and improve your self-esteem, but it is not the solution to all of life's problems.

There is yet another kind of unfulfilled promise that you may encounter upon reaching goal weight. With all the pictures of young, slender bodies in magazines, on billboards, and in the media in general, you may come to expect that weight loss will also bring a return to youth and a youthful figure. It can be quite a shock to discover you have a 43-year-old (or older) body, and not the 23-year-old bodies in the advertisements. If you have been significantly overweight for long, and especially if you have led a mostly sedentary lifestyle, you are likely to have some sagging skin and stretch marks; and without a developed muscle structure, your body might not look quite as you had expected.

In fact, losing weight is not the modern version of The Fountain of Youth. You may still not have the body you desire, even if you do reach goal weight. (There are some things you can do—you can take up weight training to reshape your muscle structure, and you can seek the help of a plastic surgeon who can usually make some skin tucks that will help some of the sagging. Also, depending on your age and your genetic inheritance, the sags may disappear by themselves with time.)

Ultimately, successful maintenance of goal weight comes down to self-acceptance—of your body as it is, of your age and the fact that you are getting older, and of who you are. This is especially difficult for women, because they have been ingrained with the notion that their body is a reflection of their value, and that aging is tantamount to obsolescence.

Even though the message of society about what weight means seems overwhelming, you can begin to cope by taking charge of your thinking. Use thought stopping when you find yourself engrossed in self-pity or self-condemnation. Change your self-talk, and practice self-acceptance in what you say to yourself about yourself.

It may help to remind yourself that the entire population is aging, and by the turn of the century, there will be more people over the age of 60 than under 60. Even now, "older" women—Jane Fonda, Raquel Welch, and others—are admired for their beauty and are setting new standards that may ultimately influence society's values. In the meantime, learn to look in the mirror and like what you see—even though the reflection might not appear on a billboard advertising cigarettes. When you can do that, you have indeed "come a long way baby!"

Control and Food

Perhaps you do just fine managing food while you are losing weight. You are a "good dieter," and feel in control while dieting. The problem begins when you reach goal weight, because you cannot or do not make the transition from dieting to eating in moderation.

Yours is a love/hate relationship with food. While dieting, you "hate" food and restrict it by exerting control. Reaching goal weight, however, redefines things. Technically you should no longer hate food, but you are afraid to let yourself enjoy it. You believe that if you allow yourself to enjoy food, the flood gates will open, and all your pent-up desire will come rushing out to consume everything in sight. Often this becomes a self-fulfilling prophecy.

The problem here really starts when restrictive dieting is the method for losing weight. On the other hand, if you have tried learning to eat in moderation, and have integrated this principle into your weight management program, this problem is less likely to crop up. But in any event, if you have difficulty with food in this way, you need to set up situations to teach yourself that you will not lose control even if you let yourself enjoy food.

Francine was nearing her goal weight for the third time, and she was well aware that her love/hate relationship with food had been the source of her difficulty in coping with success. This time she had allowed herself to try out the Principle of Moderation, and she had been relatively successful with it. Still, she was afraid that she would lose control if she ever really let herself enjoy food.

One of the practice situations she set up to teach herself that she would not lose control involved going out to dinner at a favorite restaurant with her husband. Her plan was to allow herself to enjoy and savor each bite of the dinner, but she was also to eat slowly, and to leave some food on her plate.

In addition, she was to reserve a part of her consciousness to watch the rest of herself enjoy the meal. Specifically, the "observer" in her was to notice that she was not losing control—she was not shovelling food into her mouth, she was not ordering extras of anything, she was even leaving food on the plate! The observer was to notice how the feeling of fullness increased the longer she ate, and that leaving food on the plate was easier when she was conscious of the fullness in her stomach.

Through this and other such "controlled" practice sessions, while allowing herself to enjoy food, Francine gradually overcame her fear of losing control. She also used imagery to visualize herself relaxing and enjoying food in moderation, and she developed self-talk to instruct herself in what to do and how to feel before, during, and after eating.

Finally, Francine was able to acknowledge the possibility that at some time or other she might again go temporarily out of control with food, but that this need not mean she was permanently out of control. In anticipation of this possibility, she considered ahead what steps she would take to get back on track, without resorting to defining food as fearsome or hateful. To ensure continued success, Francine had to get off the in-control/out-of-control see-saw, and develop confidence in her ability to cope effectively.

Eating Successfully

One of the most difficult problems for the person who is switching from the actively-trying-to-lose-weight phase to the maintenance phase is learning to integrate food and calories back into the daily diet. In some cases, this means adding calories back into the diet to stabilize weight at a maintenance level. In other cases it means eating "real" food instead of special diet food. In either event, this is a time that is especially frightening and fraught with problems for the person newly at goal weight.

There are several strategies for learning to eat successfully after reaching a maintenance level. One is systematically to add back calories until you reach a maintenance level of caloric intake that you then maintain. Another approach is to alternate "dieting" and eating "normally." Yet another is to establish a set of rules that guide your food choices. In this strategy, you do not follow a "diet" per se; rather the "eating structure" guides your choices. The key, in this case, is to learn to use moderation.

Systematically Adding Back Calories

Systematically adding back calories until a maintenance level is reached is a standard technique for stabilizing weight at a particular level. Once you reach the weight you want (or after going a pound or two below it), add back some additional calories in increments of 50 or 100 a day for the first week. (For instance, if you have been limiting your eating to 1,000 calories per day, increase your eating to 1,050 or 1,100 calories per day for the week.)

Weigh yourself at the end of the week to see what effect these extra calories are having. Then add another 50 or 100 calories the following week and each subsequent week until your weight stabilizes.

It is especially important at this time to keep a careful record of exactly what you are eating and how many calories you are adding to your normal fare. Sometimes there is an initial jump in weight when you start adding back calories. Don't let this frighten you. Changes in fluid retention may be contributing. Just maintain your intake at the new caloric level until things stabilize.

When John got to his maintenance goal weight, he wanted to know why he couldn't immediately go from 1200 calories a day to what (according to the formulas for calculating caloric need) should be his maintenance calorie level of 2200 to 2400, instead of adding back calories a little at a time.

If he had jumped up to this level immediately, the chances are he would have gained weight, because his body was poised to store calories. Even modest caloric restriction can prime the body to turn extra calories into stored fat. Adding back calories slowly gives the body a chance to adjust to the increased caloric intake without overcompensating and storing fat. Eventually John did move up to the higher level, but it had to be done gradually.

Furthermore, there is now evidence that some people who lose weight have to consume fewer calories (at least for a while) than lean people of the same weight and energy level just to maintain their new body weight. This is particularly true for those who have a family history of obesity or who are older. For these people to maintain weight successfully, drastic changes in diet and exercise are required, but it is possible.

Alternating Restriction and "Normal" Eating

For some people, an alternative strategy for maintaining goal weight is to follow a pattern of eating carefully (i.e., "dieting") during the week, and letting themselves eat "normally" on weekends—that is, not worrying about what they eat. In fact, "not worrying about weight" is not the eating style of most normal weight people; it is more likely that of those who will develop a weight problem in the future.

The notion that normal weight people don't watch what they eat is a fantasy. Of course, there are a few people who don't ever think about what they eat; their bodies just naturally remain lean. These "naturally thin" people have a metabolism or biochemical situation that mediates against weight gain.

Most people of normal weight fall into one of two other categories— "maintained normals," who are relatively conscious about what they eat and/ or who exercise regularly, and "delayed overweights," who are presently normal weight and don't think about what they eat, but whose eating style and exercise habits will eventually produce a weight problem. The eating style that produces long-term normal weight, is moderation.

Establishing an "Eating Structure"

An alternative to following a specific diet is to create for yourself a set of guidelines that structure your food choices. Such an "eating structure" may begin initially as a diet, but it does not require counting calories. Rather, this method involves establishing for yourself a set of choices that govern what or how you may eat at meals, snacks, and special occasions.

So, for breakfast, you might decide that you can choose between dry cereal with nonfat milk, or a poached egg on a half a muffin, or cut-up fruit with yogurt. You might build in some flexibility by adding that on one weekend day you might allow yourself pancakes or french toast. On vacations or special occasions, you might allow yourself free choice practiced in moderation (more on moderation shortly).

A similar set of decisions is established for other meals and eating occasions. By doing so, you don't find yourself wondering, "What would I like for breakfast?" only to end up with greasy bacon and eggs too often. The choices you set for yourself are healthy ones; you don't have to count calories; and you practice moderation.

Moderation means that no food is forbidden or decreed "illegal," but it also means a healthy balance, in favor of the "healthy" choices. To do this successfully and make moderation a life habit usually requires reeducating your taste buds and reprogramming your food preferences. Time and persistence are your best allies here.

The more you make low-sodium choices, for example, the less you will like the taste of salt. Self-talk helps too. Tell yourself you don't really enjoy or don't really want a particular food, and that you really do want an alternative choice. Define yourself in particular ways—"I don't eat red meat; I prefer chicken or fish."

Alter your preferences in stages. First move from fatty red meat choices to leaner meat choices, then to fewer choices of any meat, and then to choices involving more legumes and complex carbohydrates. Allow yourself occasional deviations if you want, but let moderation be your guiding principle.

Maintaining Vigilance and Self-Awareness

Successful maintainers differ from those who regain the weight they lost in that they are able to maintain adequate vigilance and self-awareness without becoming obsessed with dieting and eating. In particular, succeeders have a particular kind of internal alarm that sends a signal when weight is getting out of hand. Not only does the succeeder pay attention to her own behavior, she notices the consequences of this behavior sooner than does the unsuccessful maintainer.

The successful maintainer usually has a "3-lb. alarm." That is, when her weight is about three pounds over goal, she takes immediate action. When she has an eating slip, she takes corrective action the next day at the latest—compensating by reducing intake somewhat and/or doing some additional exercise.

The person who tends to regain, on the other hand, has an alarm that tends to go off much later—usually after significant damage is done. In effect she seems not to notice an eating indiscretion, and she avoids feedback (such as getting on the scale) that tells her things are going awry. It is not until she has regained ten or 20 pounds or more that she takes notice, and then she may panic. As a result, she sets herself up for the yo-yo cycle of weight loss and regain.

To maintain success, you must develop a level of vigilance and self-awareness that will prompt corrective action when it will be most beneficial—which is usually sooner than later. This means periodically weighing yourself, or having some other means of judging how well you are maintaining your weight.

When certain clothes no longer fit right, you can be sure something is happening with your weight. You need to keep mental tabs on your eating and exercise habits. Periodically writing down what you eat and the circumstances surrounding your eating—what led you to eat what you ate, and how you felt and what you did afterwards—can also be helpful in interrupting a return to bad eating habits.

Finding "True" Success

Reaching goal weight is not really success. Joan Beall, who manages the Weight Watchers program in Virginia Beach, Virginia, and who works with lecturers to help them maintain their goal weight, comments, "I've seen many people reach goal weight, but few of them truly succeed. Reaching goal weight is really pseudo-success. Making the mental switch that allows you to stay at goal weight is the secret of true success. I personally believe that this happens when the person begins the process of personal growth that is characterized by developing greater awareness of herself and the aspects of her life."

Successful weight loss involves self-discovery as well as self-nurturing. The truth is that losing weight is a selfcentered preoccupation, and that's as it should be. But the paradox is that success in *maintaining* goal weight requires some refocusing.

Although it is necessary to maintain enough vigilance to take corrective action when necessary, the successful maintenance phase ultimately requires getting in touch with and creating for yourself interests and projects that will provide you with a sense of self-confidence and personal satisfaction. It may mean doing the work it takes to heal old wounds—that is, getting the help of a psychotherapist or joining an appropriate self-help group.

Successful maintenance also involves a question of balance—between meeting your own needs, and meeting the needs of others; between attending to your personal situation, and putting energy into things outside yourself. It requires making the basic changes that have already been discussed—making exercise a permanent part of your lifestyle, keeping total calories and especially fat calories low, and continuing to get support for your new eating and behavior changes.

From Victimization to Empowerment

When Oprah declared, "I'll never diet again," she echoed the frustration of hundreds of thousands of dieters who have tried and failed to take weight off and keep it off. Like Oprah, some have surrendered to being a victim—of their genes, their biology, their fat cells, their metabolism, their addiction, their willpower, or their personal history. Society, and even some members of the helping professions, has alternately attributed the dieter's weight problem to a personality problem, to immorality, or to a "disease."

Some of these explanations may contain a kernel of truth, but all of them fail to take into account the human spirit, and what can happen when a person believes in himself or herself. Over and over again, scientific inquiry has demonstrated that believing you can make a difference increases your power to do so, whereas believing that what you do makes no difference produces feelings of helplessness and hopelessness, leading ultimately to failure.

Despite the fact that the odds are against keeping the weight off, there are people who have managed to lose weight and keep it off permanently. Most certainly they do the things that research shows make the difference— they exercise, they watch what they eat, they get continued support, they manage themselves and their relationships so that they get sufficient satisfaction and joy out of life. But they do one more thing that is critically important —they believe in themselves.

Where there are obstacles, these successful maintainers see opportunities to learn and overcome. Where others see failure, they find hope. Where some discount or dismiss, they notice progress. They make opportunities to nurture themselves, to soothe themselves, and to heal themselves. They practice acceptance—of themselves and others. They stand up for their rights, while respecting the rights of others.

You too must believe in yourself if you are to succeed in keeping off the weight you've lost. It will take a change in your thinking. You need to flip the mental switch from thinking of yourself as a person who is always struggling with a weight problem, to that of a person who has every thing it takes to be a winner—to succeed in keeping off the weight, now that you've lost it.

Appendix A

Self-Help Clearinghouses

Arizona

Rainy Day People Clearinghouse of Self-Help Support Groups (in development). (602) 840–1029, P.O. Box 472, Scottsdale, AZ 85252. Ms. Pat Becker, founder and director.

California

Self-Help Center. 1–800–222–LINK or (213) 825–1799, U.C.L.A., 405 Hilgard Avenue, Los Angeles, CA 90024. Fran Dory, Director. Provides information on other affiliated self-help clearinghouses in the state, to include those such as:

Northern Region Self-Help Center. (916) 456–2070, Mental Health Assn., 8912 Volunteer Lane, Sacramento, CA 95819. Ms. Pat Camper, Coordinator.

Bay Area Self-Help Center. (415) 921–4401, Mental Health Assn., 2398 Pine Street, San Francisco, CA 94115. Duff Axsom, Coordinator.

Central Region Self-Help Center. (209) 723–8861, Merced County Dept. of Mental Health, 650 West 19th Street, Merced, CA 95341. Nancy Silva, Coordinator.

Southern Self-Help Center. (619) 298–3152, Mental Health Assn., 3958 Third Avenue, San Diego, CA 92103. Sandra Driscoll, Coordinator.

Connecticut

Self-Help/Mutual Support Network. (203) 789–7645, Consultation Center, 19 Howe Street, New Haven, CT 06511. Vicki Spiro Smith, Director.

Illinois

Self-Help Center. 1–800–322–MASH (in Illinois only) or (312) 328–0470, 1600 Dodge Avenue, Suite S-122, Evanston, IL 60201. Daryl Isenberg, Director.

Self-Help Center. (312) 328–0470, Family Service of Champaign County, 405 South State Street, Champaign, IL 61820. Janine Giese-Davis, Coordinator.

Iowa

Self-Help Clearinghouse. 1–800–383–4777 (from within Iowa only), (515) 576–5870; Iowa Pilot Parents, Inc., 33 North 12th Street, Fort Dodge, IA 50501. Carla Lawson, Director.

Kansas

Self-Help Network. 1–800–445–0116 (in Kansas only) or (316) 689–3170, Campus Box 34, Wichita State University, Wichita, KS 67208-1595. David Gleason, Director.

Massachusetts

Clearinghouse of Mutual Help Groups. (413) 545–2313, Massachusetts Cooperative Extension, 113 Skinner Hall, University of Massachusetts, Amherst, MA 01003. Warren Schumacher, Director.

Michigan

Self-Help Clearinghouse. (517) 484–7373, 1–800–752–5858 (in Michigan only), Michigan Protection & Advocacy Service, 109 West Michigan Avenue, Suite 900, Lansing, MI 48933. Ms. Toni Young, Coordinator.

Center for Self-Help. 1–800–336–0341 (in Michigan only) (616) 925–0594, Riverwood Center, 1485 Highway M-139, Benton Harbor, MI 49022. Ms. Pat Friend, Director.

Minnesota

First Call for Help. (612) 224–1133 for referrals, administrative number is 291–8427; 166 East 4th Street, St. Paul, MN 55104. Diane Faulds, Coordinator.

Missouri

The Support Group Clearinghouse. (816) 561–HELP; Kansas City Assn. for Mental Health, 706 W. 42nd St., Kansas City, MO 64111. Becky Brozovich, Coordinator.

Nebraska

Self-Help Information Services. (402) 476–9668, 1601 Euclid Avenue, Lincoln, NE 68502. Barbara Fox, Director.

New Jersey

Self-Help Clearinghouse. 1–800–367–6274 (in New Jersey only), (201) 625–9565, TDD (201) 625–9053, St. Clares-Riverside Medical Center, Pocono Road, Denville, NJ 07834. Edward J. Madara, Director.

New York

New York State Self-Help Clearinghouse. (518) 442–5337, at SUNY School of Social Welfare, Richardson Hall, 135 Western Avenue, Albany, NY 12222. Linda Rotering, Director. The Clearinghouse provides information on many additional local clearinghouses in the state (upstate) other than the following ones:

New York City Self-Help Clearinghouse. (718) 596–6000, P.O. Box 022812, Brooklyn, NY 11202. Marilyn Ng-A-Qui, Director.

Brooklyn Self-Help Clearinghouse. (718) 834–7341, 934–7373, 30 Third Avenue, Brooklyn, NY 11217. Rose Langfelder, Director.

Westchester Self-Help Clearinghouse. (914) 347–3620, Westchester Community College, 75 Grasslands Road, Valhalla, NY 10595. Leslie Borck, Director.

Long Island Self-Help Clearinghouse. (516) 348–3030, New York Institute of Technology, Central Islip Campus, Central Islip, NY 11722. Pat Verdino, Director.

North Carolina

Supportworks. (Serving greater Mecklenberg area), (704) 331–9500, 1012 Kings Drive, Suite 923, Charlotte, NC 28283. Joal Fischer, Director.

Oregon

Northwest Regional Self-Help Clearinghouse. (502) 222–5555, (503) 225–9360 admin.; 718 W. Burnside Avenue, Portland, OR 97209. Judy Hadley, Coordinator.

Pennsylvania

Self-Help Group Network of the Pittsburgh Area. (412) 261–5363, 1323 Forbes Avenue, Pittsburgh, PA 15219. Betty Hepner, Coordinator.

Self-Help Information & Networking Exchange. (717) 961–1234; SHINE, Voluntary Action Center of Northeast Pennsylvania, 225 N. Washington Avenue, Park Plaza, Lower Level, Scranton, PA 18503. Gail Bauer, Director.

Philadelphia Clearinghouse. (Self-help clearinghouse planned), (215) 482–4316, c/o Self-Help Institute, 462 Monastery Avenue, Philadelphia, PA 19128. Gwen Olitsky, Contact Person.

Rhode Island

The Support Group Helpline. (401) 277–2231, Rhode Island Dept. of Health, Cannon Building, Davis Street, Providence, RI 02908. Deborah Reavey, Contact Person.

South Carolina

Midland Area Support Group Network. (803) 791–9227 I&R; (803) 791–2049 administrative; Lexington Medical Center, 2720 Sunset Boulevard, West Columbia, SC 29169. Mary Burton, Director.

Tennessee

Support Group Clearinghouse. (615) 584–6736, Mental Health Assn. of Knox County, 6712 Kingston Pike #203, Knoxville, TN 37919. Judy Balloff, Coordinator.

Texas

Texas Self-Help Clearinghouse. (512) 476–0611, Mental Health Assn. in Texas, 1111 W. 24 Street, Austin, TX 78705. Several other clearinghouses in Texas include:

Dallas Self-Help Clearinghouse. (214) 871–2420, Mental Health Assn., 2500 Maple Avenue, Dallas, TX 75201-1998. Carol Madison, Director.

Houston Area Self-Help Clearinghouse. Houston & Harris counties (713) 523–8963, Mental Health Assn., 221 Norfolk, Houston, TX 77098. Dianne Long, Coordinator.

San Antonio Self-Help Clearinghouse. (512) 826–2288, Mental Health Assn., 1407 North Main, San Antonio, TX 78212.

Washington, D.C.

Self-Help Clearinghouse of Greater Washington. (703) 536–4100, Mental Health Assn., 100 N. Washington Street, Falls Church, VA 22046. Lisa Saisselin, Coordinator.

National Information—U.S.

American Self-Help Clearinghouse. 1–800–367–6274 (in New Jersey only), (201) 625–9565, TDD (201) 625–9053, St. Clares-Riverside Medical Center, Pocono Road, Denville, NJ 07834. Edward J. Madara, Director.

National Self-Help Clearinghouse. (212) 642–2944, City University of New York Graduate Center, Room 620, 25 West 43rd Street, New York, NY 10036. Frank Riessman, Director.

Self-Help Center. (312) 328–0470, 1600 Dodge Avenue, Suite S-122, Evanston, IL 60201. Daryl Isenberg, Director.

Canada

Canadian Council on Social Development. (613) 728–1865, P.O. Box 3505, Station C, Ottawa, Ontario, Canada K1Y 4G1. Self-help promotional activities, to include national newsletter.

Calgary

Family Life Education Council. (403) 262–1117, 233 12th Avenue SW, Calgary, Alberta, Canada T2R OG9. Sonia Eisler, Executive Director.

Nova Scotia

The Self-Help Connection. (902) 422–5831, 5739 Inglis Street, Halifax, Nova Scotia, Canada B3H 1K5. Margot Clarke, Coordinator.

Sasketchewan

Self-Help Development Unit. (306) 652–7817, 410 Cumberland Avenue North, Sakatoon, Saskatchewan, Canada S7M 1M6. Richard Wollert, Director.

Toronto

Self-Help Clearinghouse of Metro. Toronto. (416) 487–4355, 40 Orchard View Boulevard, Suite 215, Toronto, Ontario, Canada M4R 1B9. Lori Kociol, Director.

Winnipeg

Self-Help Resource Clearinghouse. (204) 589–5500 or 633–5955, NorWest Coop & Health Center, 103-61 Tyndall Avenue, Winnipeg, Manitoba, Canada R2X 2T4.

Overseas

Australia

Western Institute of Self-Help. (09) 383–3188, 80 Railway Street, Cottesloe, 6011, Western Australia.

Europe

International Information Centre on Self-Help and Health. E. Van Evenstraat 2C, B-3000 Leuven, Belgium. Provides information on clearinghouses and projects throughout Europe. Jan Branckaerts, Director.

England

National Self-Help Support Centre. NCVO, 26 Bedford Square, London, England WC1B 2HU. Mai Wann, Director.

Germany

National Kontakt und Informationsstelle zur Amregung & Unterstutzung von Selbsthilfegruppen. Albrecth-Achilles-Strasse 65, D-1000 Berlin 31. Klaus Balke, Director.

Israel

Self-Help Clearinghouse. Phone 661231, American Jewish Joint Distribution Committee, Inc., J.D.C. Hill, Jersalem, Israel 91034. Martha Ramon, Director.

Japan

Society for Study of Self-Help Groups. Dept of Social Welfare, Faculty of Humanities, Sophia University, 7-1 Kiolcho, Chiyoda-ky, Tokyo 102, Japan. Tomofumi Oka, Director.

Appendix B

Resource Organizations

Eating Disorders

American Anorexia/Bulimia Association, Inc.
133 Cedar Lane
Teaneck, New Jersey 07666
201–836–1800

National Association of Anorexia Nervosa and Associated Disorders
P.O. Box 271
Highland Park, Illinois 60035
708–831–3438

Overeaters Anonymous—National Office
4025 Spencer Street, Suite 203
Torrance, California 90504
213–542–8363

O-Anon
Check local listings.

Child Abuse (physical and sexual)

Adults Molested as Children United (AMACU)
P.O. Box 952
San Jose, California 95108
408–280–5055

Incest Survivors Anonymous (ISA)
P.O. Box 5613
Long Beach, California 90805
213–422–1632

Incest Survivors Resource Network, International, Inc.
P.O. Box 911
Hicksville, New York 11802
516–935–3031

National Child Abuse Hotline
Childhelp USA
P.O. Box 630
Hollywood, California 90028
800–4–A–CHILD (800–422–4453)

Parents Anonymous—National Office
6733 South Sepulveda Boulevard, Suite 270
Los Angeles, California 90045
800–421–0353

Survivors of Incest Gaining Health (SIGH)
20 West Adams, Suite 2015
Chicago, Illinois 60606

Victims Anonymous (VA)
9514–9 Roseda Boulevard #607
Northridge, California 91324
818–993–1139

Victims of Incest Can Emerge Survivors (V.O.I.C.E.S.) in Action
P.O. Box 148309
Chicago, Illinois 60614
312–327–1500

Alcoholism and the Family

Al-Anon Family Group Headquarters
1372 Broadway (at 38th Street), 7th Floor
New York, New York 10018
800–245–4656
212–302–7240 (in New York area)

Alateen
Call Al-Anon (cited above).

Alcoholics Anonymous—General Services Office (AA)
468 Park Avenue South
New York, New York 10016
212–686–1100

Alcoholics Anonymous World Services (AA)
P.O. Box 459, Grand Central Station
New York, New York 10163
212–686–1100

Children of Alcoholics Foundation
200 Park Avenue, 31st Floor
New York, New York 10166
212–949–1404

National Association of Children of Alcoholics (NACOA)
31706 Coast Highway
South Laguna, California 92677
714–499–3889

Rational Recovery Systems[1] (RR)
P.O. Box 800
Lotus, California 95651
916–621–4374

Recovery, Inc.[2]
802 North Dearborn Street
Chicago, Illinois 60610
312–337–5661
510–351–2540

Secular Organization for Sobriety (SOS)
(also known as Save Our Selves)
P.O. Box 5
Buffalo, New York 14215
716–834–2922

Women for Sobriety & Men for Sobriety (WFS and MFS[3])
P.O. Box 618
Quakertown, PA 18915
215–536–8026
800–333–1606

---

[1] There is a separate, unrelated organization called "Rational Recovery" that operates in the Ft. Lauderdale, Florida, area.

[2] Self-help for nervous symptoms and fears.

[3] The meetings for these two groups operate separately.

Drug Addiction

American Atheist Addiction Recovery Groups (AAARG)
2344 South Broadway
Denver, Colorado 80210
303–722–1525

Cocaine Anonymous—National Office
P.O. Box 1367
Culver City, California 90232
213–559–5833

Drugs Anonymous
Look for groups in your area.

Narcotics Anonymous—World Services Office (NA)
P.O. Box 9999
Van Nuys, California 91409
818–780–3951

Nar-Anon
Check local listings.

National Cocaine Abuse Hotline
800–COCAINE (800–262–2463)

National Institute of Drug Abuse (NIDA)
Parklawn Building, 5600 Fishers Lane
Rockville, Maryland 20852
Information Office: 301–443–6245
          For Help: 800–662–HELP (800–662–4357)
          For Employers: 800–843–4971
          For Literature: National Clearinghouse for Information
                         P.O. Box 416
                         Kensington, Maryland 20895

Compulsive Gambling

Gamblers Anonymous
National Council on Compulsive Gambling
444 West 56th Street, Room 3207S
New York, New York 10019
212–765–3833

GamAnon
Check local listings.

Compulsive Spending

Debtors Anonymous
Check local area for groups, or for Shopaholic groups.

Spender Menders
Check local listings.

Nervous Symptoms, Fears, and Other Emotions

Emotions Anonymous
Check local listings.

Recovery, Inc.
802 North Dearborn Street
Chicago, Illinois 60610
312–337–5661
510–351–2540

Sex Addiction and the Family

Sex Addicts Anonymous (SAA)
P.O. Box 3038
Minneapolis, Minnesota 55403
612–871–1520

Codependents of Sexual Addicts (COSA)
P.O. Box 14537
Minneapolis, Minnesota 55414

Sexaholics Anonymous (SA)
P.O. Box 300
Simi Valley, California 93062
818–704–9854

S-Anon
P.O. Box 5117
Sherman Oaks, California 91413
818–990–6910

Sex and Love Addicts Anonymous (SLAA)
Augustine Fellowship
P.O. Box 119
New Town Branch
Boston, Massachusetts 02258

National Association on Sex Addiction Problems
800–622–9494

Sexually Transmitted Diseases

VD National Hotline
1–800–227–8922
1–800–982–5883 (in California)

Herpes Resource Center
415–328–7710

American Social Health Association
260 Sheridan Avenue, Suite 307
Palo Alto, California 94306

National AIDS Hotline
800–342–AIDS (800–342–2437)

Index

Made in the USA
Lexington, KY
12 January 2011